Fifty Cases *of* Peripheral Vascular Interventions

FIFTY CASES *of*

PERIPHERAL

VASCULAR

INTERVENTIONS

Edited by

Christopher J White MD

Chairman
Department of Cardiology
Ochsner Heart and Vascular Institute
New Orleans LA
USA

MARTIN DUNITZ

2002 Martin Dunitz Ltd, a member of the Taylor & Francis Group

First published in the United Kingdom in 2002 by Martin Dunitz Ltd, The Livery House, 7-9 Pratt Street, London NW1 0AE

Tel: +44 (0) 20 7482 2202
Fax: +44 (0) 20 7267 0159
E-mail: info@dunitz.co.uk
Webiste: http://www.dunitz.co.uk

A CIP record for this book is available from the British Library.

ISBN 1-84184-098-X

Although every effort has been made to ensure that all owners of copyright material have been acknowledged in this publication, we would be glad to acknowledge in subsequent reprints or editions any omissions brought to our attention.

Distributed in the USA by
Fulfilment Center
Taylor & Francis
7625 Empire Drive
Florence, KY 41042, USA
Toll Free Tel.: +1 800 634 7064
E-mail: cserve@routledge_ny.com

Distributed in Canada by
Taylor & Francis
74 Rolark Drive
Scarborough, Ontario M1R 4G2, Canada
Toll Free Tel.: +1 877 226 2237
E-mail: tal_fran@istar.ca

Distributed in the rest of the world by
ITPS Limited
Cheriton House
North Way
Andover,
Hampshire SP10 5BE
UK
Tel.: +44 (0)1264 332424
E-mail: reception@itps.co.uk

Composition by 🅣Tek-Art

Printed and Bound in Great Britain by Biddles Ltd, Guildford and King's Lynn

To Janet, the love of my life;
and the lights of my life, my four wonderful children,
Casey, Jimmy, Jordan and Samantha

CONTENTS

Section IV: Aorto-iliac lower extremity interventions

List of Contributors

William B Abernathy MD
St Elizabeth's Medical Center,
Brighton MA 02135,
USA.

Nadim Al-Mubarak MD
The Lenox Hill Heart and Vascular
Institute,
New York City NY 10021,
USA.

Ramin Alimard MD
Medical College of Virginia,
Richmond VA 23298,
USA.

Jose Norberto Allende MD
Unidad CardioVascular-Sanatorio
Allende-Cordoba 5000,
Argentina.

Gary M Ansel MD
Director,
Peripheral Vascular Intervention,
Riverside Methodist Hospital,
MidOhio Cardiology Consultants,
MidWest Cardiology Research
Foundation,
Columbus OH 43214,
Assistant Clinical Professor of
Medicine,
Medical College of Toledo,
Toledo OH
USA.

J Michael Bacharach MD
North Central Heart Institute,
Sioux Falls SD 57108,
USA.

Christopher Bajzer MD
Cleveland Clinic Foundation,
Cleveland OH 44195,
USA.

Laura Berke MD
St Elizabeth's Medical Center,
Brighton MA 02135,
USA.

Giancarlo Biamino MD
Center for Cardiology and Vascular
Intervention,
22763 Hamburg,
Germany.

Alan S Boulos MD
Department of Neurosurgery,
University of New York at Buffalo,
Buffalo NY 14209,
USA.

Simon Chough MD
Pittsburgh Vascular Institute,
Pittsburgh PA, USA.

Tyrone J Collins MD
Department of Cardiology,
Ochsner Heart and Vascular Institute,
New Orleans LA,
USA.

Antonio Colombo MD
Director,
Cardiac Catheterization Laboratory,
Centro Cuore Columbus,
20129 Milano,
Director, Invasive Cardiology,
San Raffaele,
20132 Milano, Italy,
Director, Investigational Angioplasty,
Lenox Hill Hospital,
New York NY 10021,
USA.

Michael J Cowley MD
Medical College of Virginia,
Richmond VA 23298,
USA.

Frank J Criado MD FACS
Director,
Center for Vascular Intervention,
Chief,
Division of Vascular Surgery,
Union Memorial Hospital,
Baltimore MD 21218,
USA.

Rajesh M Dave MD
Ohio Heart Health Center,
Cincinnati OH 45219,
USA.

Louis DePaolo MD
Department of Surgery,
Mount Sinai School of Medicine,
New York NY 10029,
USA.

Edward B Diethrich MD
Medical Director,
Arizona Health Institute,
Phoenix AZ 85006,
USA.

Andrew C Eisenhauer MD
Brigham & Womens Hospital,
Boston MA 02115,
USA.

Gustav R Eles MD
Pittsburgh Vascular Institute,
Pittsburgh PA,
USA.

Peter Fail MD
Cardiovascular Institute of the South,
Houma LA 70361,
USA.

Joseph M Garasic MD
Brigham & Womens Hospital,
Boston MA 02115,
USA.

Thomas P Gehrig MD
Duke University Medical Center,
Durham NC 27710,
USA.

D Luke Glancy MD
Section of Cardiology,
Department of Medicine,
Louisiana State University Health
Sciences Center,
New Orleans LA 70112,
USA.

Evelyne Goudreau MD
Medical College of Virginia,
Richmond VA 23298,
USA.

Manohar Gowda MD
MidAmerica Heart Institute,
Kansas City MO 64111,
USA.

Lee R Guterman MD
Department of Neurosurgery,
University of New York at Buffalo,
Buffalo NY 14209,
USA.

Isabelle Henry MD
Maladie du Coeur et des Vaisseaux –
Cardiologie Interventionelle,
54000 Nancy,
France.

Michel Henry MD
Maladie du Coeur et des Vaisseaux –
Cardiologie Interventionelle,
54000 Nancy,
France.

James Hermiller MD
Director of Cardiac Cath Labs,
St Vincent Hospital,
Indianapolis,
IN 46062,
USA.

Richard R Heuser MD FACC FACP
Director of Research,
St. Lukes Medical Center,
Phoenix AZ 85006,
USA.

Larry H Hollier MD
Department of Surgery,
Mount Sinai School of Medicine,
New York NY 10029,
USA.

L Nelson Hopkins MD
Department of Neurosurgery,
University of New York at Buffalo,
Buffalo NY 14209,
USA.

Jeffrey M Isner MD
St Elizabeth's Medical Center,
Boston MA 02135,
USA.

Suresh P Jain MD
Section of Cardiology,
Department of Medicine,
Louisiana State University Health
Sciences Center,
New Orleans LA 70112,
USA.

J Stephen Jenkins MD
Department of Cardiology,
Ochsner Heart and Vascular Institute,
New Orleans LA 70121,
USA.

Christoph Kalka MD
St Elizabeth's Medical Center,
Brighton MA 02135,
USA.

Bahij N Khuri MD
Section of Cardiology,
Department of Medicine,
Louisiana State University Health
Sciences Center,
New Orleans LA 70112,
USA.

Zvonimir Krajcer MD
Department of Cardiology,
Texas Heart Institute / St Luke's
Episcopal Hospital,
Houston TX 77030,
USA.

Paul Kramer MD
Kramer and Crouse Cardiology PC,
MidAmerica Heart Institute,
Saint Luke's Hospital of Kansas City,
Kansas City MO 64111,
USA.

John Laird MD
Director,
Peripheral Vascular Interventions,
Cardiovascular Research Institute,
Washington Hospital Center,
Washington DC 20010,
USA.

David T Lee MD
Interventional Cardiologist,
Michigan Cardiovascular Institute,
Saginaw MI 48604,
USA.

James T Lee MD
Harbor-UCLA Medical Center,
Torrance CA,
USA.

Francesco Liistro MD
Interventional Cardiologist,
Emodinamica Osdpedale San Raffaele,
20132 Milano,
Italy.

Jane M Lingelbach MD
Center for Vascular Intervention,
Union Memorial Hospital,
Baltimore MD 21218,
USA.

Audrey Loeb MD
MidAmerica Heart Institute,
Kansas City MO 64111,
USA.

Hugo Francisco Londero MD FSCAI
Unidad CardioVascular-Sanatorio
Allende-Cordoba 5000,
Argentina.

Demetrius K Lopes MD
Department of Neurosurgery,
University of New York at Buffalo,
Buffalo NY 14209,
USA.

Michael L Marin MD
Director,
Endovascular Surgical Development,
Mt Sinai Medical Center,
New York NY 10029,
USA.

Germano Melissano MD
Department of Vascular Surgery,
Osdpedale San Raffaele,
20132 Milano,
Italy.

Samuel R Money MD
Ochsner Clinic,
New Orleans LA 70121,
USA.

Nicholas J Morrisey MD
Department of Surgery,
Mount Sinai School of Medicine,
New York NY 10029,
USA.

Debabrata Mukherjee MD
Department of Cardiovascular
Medicine,
Cleveland Clinic Foundation,
Cleveland OH 44195,
USA.

Fadi Naddour MD
Section of Cardiology,
Department of Medicine,
Louisiana State University Health
Sciences Center,
New Orleans LA 70112,
USA.

Francisco Eduardo Paoletti MD
Unidad CardioVascular-Sanatorio
Allende-Cordoba 5000,
Argentina.

Harry R Phillips MD
Duke University Medical Center,
Durham NC 27710,
USA.

Guy N Piegari MD
BerksCardiologists Ltd,
Reading PA 19604,
USA.

Venkatesh Ramaiah MD
Arizona Health Institute,
Phoenix AZ 85006,
USA.

Stephen R Ramee MD
Department of Cardiology,
Ochsner Heart and Vascular Institute,
New Orleans LA 70121,
USA.

Andrew J Ringer MD
Department of Neurosurgery,
University of New York at Buffalo,
Buffalo NY 14209,
USA.

Mark A Robbins MD
Department of Cardiovascular
Medicine,
Cleveland Clinic Foundation,
Cleveland OH 44195,
USA.

Julio A Rodriguez MD
Arizona Health Institute,
Phoenix AZ 85006,
USA.

Kenneth Rosenfield MD
St Elizabeth's Medical Center,
Brighton MA 02135,
USA.

Gary S Roubin MD, PhD
Director, Endovascular Services,
The Lenox Hill Heart and Vascular
Institute,
New York City NY 10021,
USA.

Sumeet Sachdev MD
Ohio Heart Health Center,
Cincinnati OH 45219,
USA.

Robert D Safian MD
Director,
Interventional Cardiology,
William Beaumont Hospital,
Royal Oak MI 48324,
USA.

Aditya K Samal MD
Department of Cardiology,
Ochsner Heart and Vascular Institute,
New Orleans LA,
USA.

Thomas M Shimshak MD
The Lindner Center for
Cardiovascular Research and
Education, and The Christ Hospital,
Cincinnati OH 45219,
USA.

Jose A Silva MD
Department of Cardiology,
Ochsner Heart and Vascular Institute,
Ochsner Slidell Clinic,
Slidell LA 70451,
USA.

Richard W Smalling MD PhD
Memorial Hermann Heart Center,
The University of Texas Medical
School at Houston,
Houston TX,
USA.

S Jody Stagg III MD
Director,
Peripheral Interventions,
Cardiovascular Institute of the South
Houma LA 70361,
USA.

Rajesh Subramanian MD
Department of Cardiology,
Ochsner Heart and Vascular Institute,
New Orleans LA,
USA.

Charles Thompson MD
Arizona Health Institute,
Phoenix AZ 85006,
USA.

Peter R Vale MD
St Elizabeth's Medical Center,
Boston MA 02135,
USA.

Craig Walker MD
Cardiovascular Institute of the South,
Houma LA 70361,
USA.

Christopher J White MD
Chairman Department of Cardiology,
Ochsner Heart and Vascular Institute,
New Orleans LA 70121,
USA.

Rodney A White MD
Harbor-UCLA Medical Center,
Torrance CA,
USA.

Patrick Whitlow MD
Cleveland Clinic Foundation,
Cleveland OH 44195,
USA.

Mark Wholey MD
Chairman,
Pittsburgh Vascular Institute,
Pittsburgh PA,
USA.

Michael H Wholey MD
University of Texas Health Service
Center,
San Antonio TX 78274,
USA.

Bruce L Wilkoff MD
Department of Cardiovascular
Medicine,
Cleveland Clinic Foundation,
Cleveland OH 44195,
USA.

Jay S Yadav MD
Director, Vascular Intervention,
Department of Cardiovascular Medicine,
Cleveland Clinic Foundation,
Cleveland OH 44195,
USA.

John W York MD
Ochsner Clinic,
New Orleans LA 70121,
USA.

John J Young MD
Ohio Heart Health Center,
Cincinnati OH 45219,
USA.

James P Zidar MD
Duke University Medical Center,
Durham NC 27710,
USA.

PREFACE

Percutaneous revascularization offers a non-surgical solution to many vascular pathologies previously treated with open surgical procedures. Interventional therapies, in general, reduce cost, morbidity and mortality of both coronary and peripheral revascularization procedures. Specifically, percutaneous peripheral vascular intervention makes revascularization procedures available to higher risk patients, often in combination with treatment of coronary lesions. The shifting paradigm in the treatment of peripheral vascular diseases from surgical to percutaneous methods has exceeded the supply of physician providers creating the need to train additional providers.

To facilitate an understanding of peripheral vascular intervention, this multi-authored book has been developed offering a broad range of case material selected for their teaching value. The cases are presented in a linear manner illustrating indications, strategic decision points and equipment selection issues made by experts in the field.

It is intended that these case studies, will serve as examples or templates for practitioners wishing to expand their fund of knowledge regarding peripheral vascular intervention.

Christopher J White MD
New Orleans LA
November 2001

I CAROTID, VERTEBRAL AND SUBCLAVIAN INTERVENTIONS

CASE 1: CAROTID STENT PLACEMENT WITH ABCIXIMAB

Christopher J White

Background

A 77-year-old man with inoperable three-vessel coronary disease, lifestyle-limiting angina pectoris and compensated congestive heart failure suffered a cerebrovascular event manifested by a left-sided hemiparesis 1 month before presentation. Over the past month, he has recovered nicely with only mild weakness of the left arm and leg remaining. Carotid duplex examination demonstrated a stenosis of more than 80% of the right internal carotid artery and occlusion of the left internal carotid artery. His current antiplatelet regimen included 325 mg aspirin/day. Clopidogrel (Plavix) 75 mg/day was started 1 week before the planned procedure. The indication for carotid revascularization was the patient's high risk of a cerebrovascular ischemic event with a high-grade symptomatic lesion as the sole remaining carotid artery. The indication for carotid stent placement versus surgical therapy was the patient's severe co-morbidity of ischemic heart disease and contralateral carotid occlusion, placing him in a high-risk surgical subgroup.

Procedure

The patient received no sedatives as premedication. A 6 Fr sheath was placed in the right common femoral artery. An arch aortogram and four-vessel carotid and vertebral angiography with intracerebral views were performed with a pigtail and a 125-cm-long 6 Fr JR-4 catheter. Baseline angiography confirmed a 99% stenosis of the right internal carotid artery (Figure 1.1).

The 6 Fr sheath was exchanged for a 9 Fr arterial sheath. A 6000 IU bolus of heparin was given (70 IU/kg). An abciximab (Reopro: Eli Lilly, Indianapolis, IN, USA) bolus (0.25 mg/kg) was given and 12-hour infusion (0.125 mg/kg/min) was started. The long (125 cm) 6 Fr JR-4 angiographic catheter was inserted through a 9 Fr multipurpose coronary angioplasty guiding catheter and advanced to the aortic arch over an 0.035-inch guidewire. The JR-4 catheter was selectively engaged in the innominate artery. A steerable, 0.035-inch Wholey wire (Malinckrodt, St Louis, MO) was advanced to the external carotid artery and the JR-4 catheter advanced over the wire into the right common carotid artery. The 9 Fr multipurpose guiding catheter was then advanced into the right common carotid artery over the JR-4 catheter.

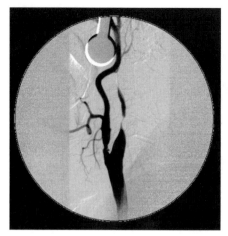

Figure 1.1 *Baseline common carotid angiogram demonstrating a subtotal occlusion of the right internal carotid artery.*

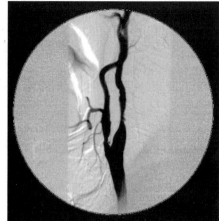

Figure 1.2 *Angiography after predilatation with a 4 mm × 40 mm balloon.*

The Wholey wire and the 6 Fr JR-4 angiographic catheter were removed and a 'roadmap' was obtained of the right internal carotid artery target lesion. An 0.018-inch Roadrunner (Cook, Bloomington, IL) guidewire was placed through a 4.0 mm × 4.0 cm Cobra (Boston Scientific Corp., Watertown, MA) balloon catheter and advanced across the lesion. The lesion was predilated with balloon inflation of 6 atm and withdrawn (Figure 1.2). The patient's blood pressure and pulse rate dropped transiently with inflation but returned to baseline without pharmacological intervention. A self-expanding 8 mm × 2 cm SMART (Cordis, Miami, FL) stent was advanced to the lesion and deployed. Post-dilation with a

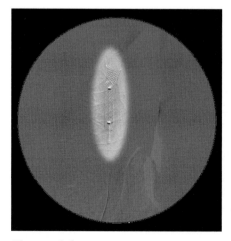

Figure 1.3 *Post-stent deployment balloon inflation.*

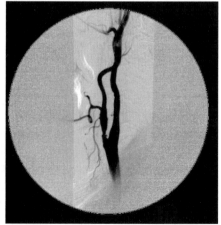

Figure 1.4 *Final angiogram with 0% residual stenosis of the right internal carotid artery.*

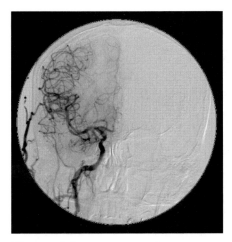

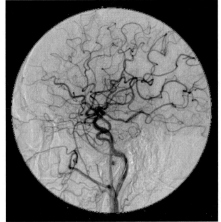

Figure 1.5 *Anterior view of the intracerebral circulation with filling of the anterior and middle cerebral arteries and unchanged from the pre-procedure images.*

Figure 1.6 *Lateral view post-stent placement of the intracerebral vessels, which is unchanged from his pre-procedure images.*

6 mm × 2 cm Opta-5 (Cordis) balloon was performed to 12 atm (Figure 1.3). Final angiography (Figure 1.4) with intracerebral views, demonstrating no distal embolization, was performed (Figure 1.5 and 1.6).

The patient's neurological examination on the table was unchanged. He was returned to the angioplasty unit for sheath removal when his activated clotting time was more than 170 seconds and discharge was planned for the next morning. His baseline neurological examination remained unchanged on routine neurology assessment after the procedure.

Commentary

This case demonstrates the use of a 9 Fr coronary guiding catheter with a 0.018-inch guidewire to deliver a self-expanding carotid stent after predilatation. It also illustrates the use of a platelet glycoprotein IIb/IIIa receptor inhibitor (abciximab) in a recently symptomatic patient. The rationale for using abiciximab is to minimize or prevent the aggregation of platelets as a source of emboli during the procedure, and perhaps to minimize the impact of distal microemboli in the cerebral circulation.

The use of IIb/IIIa glycoprotein receptor antagonists in carotid stenting remains investigational and is not accepted by all. Some argue that should an adverse event occur the patient would be more likely to hemorrhage into the brain, resulting in a fatality. Others argue that there is no proven benefit. However, given the dramatic benefit of this class of agents in the coronary circulation, it appears to be worthy of consideration, particularly in patients with recently symptomatic lesions at high risk of platelet embolization.

Case 2: Carotid stenting with emboli protection

Mark A Robbins, Jay S Yadav

Background

A 66-year-old man with a dilated cardiomyopathy (ejection fraction 12%), type 2 diabetes mellitus and left carotid endarterectomy 2 years ago now presents with deteriorating cardiac function. During the evaluation for cardiac transplantation, a carotid duplex scan revealed an estimated left internal carotid stenosis of 80–99%. Although asymptomatic, his severe carotid stenosis would have excluded him from consideration for cardiac transplantation, so, he was referred for carotid revascularization. As a result of the re-stenotic nature of the lesion and his severe cardiomyopathy, the risk for carotid endarterectomy (CEA) was increased. He was entered in the multicenter FDA-sponsored SAPPHIRE (stenting and angioplasty with protection in patients at high risk for endarterectomy) study and was randomized to carotid stenting.

Procedure

The patient was pre-treated with 300 mg clopidogrel and 325 mg aspirin the night before the procedure. His right femoral artery was entered with a 5 Fr sheath and 4000 U heparin were administered. A 5 Fr JR-4 diagnostic catheter (Cordis, Miami, FL, USA) was used for selective left and right carotid angiograms with intracranial views. The right common carotid was free of significant disease whereas the right internal carotid had no more than a 30% luminal narrowing. The right middle cerebral and anterior cerebral arteries were normal and there was cross-filling of the left anterior cerebral artery from the right carotid injection.

The distal left common carotid artery was subtotally occluded and with sluggish flow to the internal, external and cerebral vessels (Figure 2.1). The activated clotting time (ACT) before the initiation of the carotid intervention was 208 s and therefore an additional 2000 U heparin was administered, which resulted in a pre-procedural ACT of 283 s. An 8 Fr sheath was placed in the right femoral artery and the left common carotid artery was selectively engaged with an H1 8 Fr guiding catheter (Cordis).

As a result of the severity of the obstruction, the lesion was initially crossed with a 190-cm 0.014-inch Reflex wire (Cordis) and pre-dilated with 2.0 mm × 20 mm

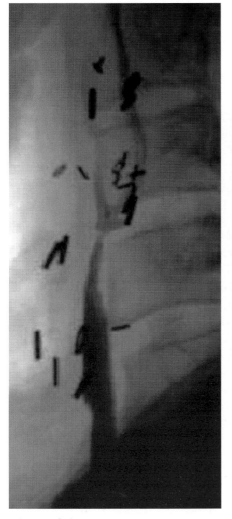

Figure 2.1 *Selective left common carotid angiography revealing a subtotal occlusion of the distal left common carotid artery.*

Figure 2.2 *Left common and internal carotid artery after the second balloon dilatation with a 2.0 mm × 20 mm Crosssail (Guidant, Temecula, CA) at 12 atm.*

Crosssail balloon (Guidant, Temecula, CA) at 4 atm for 45 s. There was significant recoil within the lesion, which required a second dilatation to 12 atm (Figure 2.2).

The Angioguard (Cordis) was then advanced though the lesion in a buddy wire fashion besides the Reflex wire without difficulty (Figure 2.3). The Reflex wire was removed and the Angioguard sheath retracted to deploy the basket in the distal internal carotid artery (ICA) (Figure 2.4). An 8 mm × 20 mm Precise (Cordis) self-expanding stent was then deployed and post-dilated with a 6 mm × 20 mm Viatrac balloon (Guidant) to 8 atm (Figure 2.5). Post-procedure

7

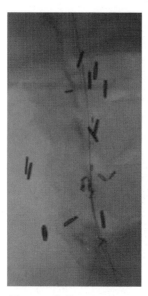

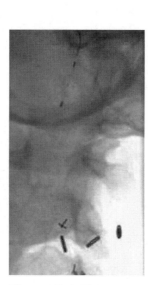

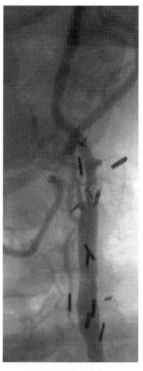

Figure 2.3 *Angiogard (Cordis, Miami, FL) device being passed through the carotid obstruction besides the Reflex wire (Cordis).*

Figure 2.4 *The Angiogard (Cordis, Miami, FL) deployed in the distal left internal carotid artery.*

Figure 2.5 *Left internal carotid artery after the deployment of an 8 mm × 20 mm Precise self-expandable stent (Cordis, Miami, FL) and post-dilatation with a 6 mm × 20 mm Viatrac balloon (Guidant, Temecula, CA).*

angiography revealed no residual stenosis. There were no neurological complications or hemodynamic instability. A 8 Fr Angio-Seal (St Jude Medical, Minnetonka, MN) was then placed in the femoral artery to obtain hemostasis.

Commentary

Distal embolization during coronary intervention is a well-established phenomenon. Platelet activation at the time of intervention, particularly with stenting, is associated with an increased risk of acute ischemic events that range from stent thrombosis to microvascular embolization and myocardial infarction. The use of abciximab, as well as other glycoprotein IIb/IIIa inhibitors has been shown dramatically to reduce the incidence of peri-procedural myocardial infarction during percutaneous coronary intervention, presumably via the prevention of microvascular embolization.

Qureshi et al[2] recently reported on the relative safety of abciximab use in a small cohort of patients in the setting of percutaneous carotid and vertebral intervention. There was no major or minor bleeding during the stenting of 13 carotid or vertebral lesions with the use of a bolus (0.25 mg/kg) and infusion (10 μg/min) of abciximab. Data from our institution on 151 consecutive patients undergoing carotid stenting, 128 with adjunctive abciximab (0.25 mg/kg bolus and 0.125 μg/kg per min infusion for 12 h) and 23 without abciximab found a significant reduction in neurological events in those treated with abciximab (8% vs 1.6%; $p=0.05$). There was one episode of delayed intracranial hemorrhage during the 30-day follow-up in the abciximab group.

The Angioguard, an emboli protection device that allows continued distal vessel visualization, may provide adequate protection without the necessity of additional antiplatelet therapy with their attendant bleeding risk, however small. If the results of SAPPHIRE and other carotid stenting trials prove that ICA stenting is as safe and effective as surgery, a randomized comparison of emboli protection versus glycoprotein IIb/IIIa inhibition versus combination therapy will be essential to determine the best strategy during percutaneous ICA intervention.

References

1. Topol EJ, Yadav JS, Recognition of the importance of embolization in atherosclerotic vascular disease. *Circulation* 2000;**101**:570–80.

2. Qureshi AI, Suri MF, Khan J, Fessler RD. Buterman LR, Hopkins LN, Abciximab as an adjunct to high-risk carotid or vertebrobasilar angioplasty: preliminary experience. *Neurosurgery* 2000;**46**:1316–24; discussion 1324–5.

3. Persson AV, Griffey EE, The natural history of total occlusion of the internal carotid artery. *Surg Clin North Am* 1985;**65**:411–16.

4. Pierce GE, Keuschkerian SM, Hermreck AS, Iliopoulos JI, Thomas JH, The risk of stroke with occlusion of the internal carotid artery. *J Vasc Surg* 1989;**9**:74–80.

5. Bornstein NM, Norris JW, Benign outcome of carotid occlusion. *Neurology* 1989;**39**:6.

6. Nicholls SC, Bergelin R, Strandness DE, Neurologic sequelae of unilateral carotid artery occlusion: immediate and late. *J Vasc Surg* 1989;**10**;542–7; discusison 547–8.

CASE 3: CAROTID ARTERY STENTING WITH DISTAL PROTECTION

Nadim Al-Mubarak, Gary S Roubin

Background

A 67-year-old man was found to have a high-grade (≥ 70%) stenosis of the right internal carotid artery during a Doppler ultrasound evaluation of asymptomatic carotid bruits.

Procedure

Access into the right common carotid artery was obtained using a 7 Fr, 90-cm-long sheath (Shuttle: Cook Inc., Bloomington, IN, USA). A single bolus of heparin (4000 units) was administered. The NeuroShield distal protection system (MedNova Inc., Gallaway, Ireland) is a temporary intravascular filtration system intended to prevent distal embolization of atheromatous material released during the carotid stenting procedures while maintaining flow (Figure 3.1). The system

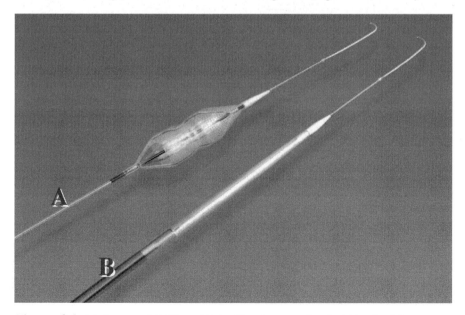

Figure 3.1 (a) An expanded filter; (b) the filter is encapsulated within the delivery sheath.

consists of three main components: the filterwire, a delivery catheter and a retrieval catheter. The filter assembly, located at the distal end of the guidewire, is sized to the selected arterial segment. The filter has four proximal entry ports and multiple distal perfusion pores which allow blood flow to the cerebral circulation while the filter is deployed. The filtration element contains a pre-shaped nitinol expansion system which assists in filter deployment and the apposition to the arterial wall.

Figure 3.2 illustrates the procedural steps of the filter application. The filterwire, encapsulated within the delivery catheter, was first advanced through

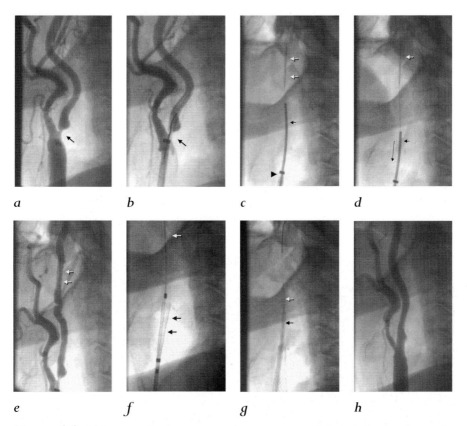

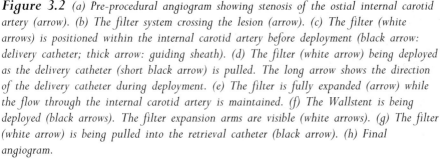

Figure 3.2 *(a) Pre-procedural angiogram showing stenosis of the ostial internal carotid artery (arrow). (b) The filter system crossing the lesion (arrow). (c) The filter (white arrows) is positioned within the internal carotid artery before deployment (black arrow: delivery catheter; thick arrow: guiding sheath). (d) The filter (white arrow) being deployed as the delivery catheter (short black arrow) is pulled. The long arrow shows the direction of the delivery catheter during deployment. (e) The filter is fully expanded (arrow) while the flow through the internal carotid artery is maintained. (f) The Wallstent is being deployed (black arrows). The filter expansion arms are visible (white arrows). (g) The filter (white arrow) is being pulled into the retrieval catheter (black arrow). (h) Final angiogram.*

11

the guiding sheath and across the target lesion. The delivery catheter was then retracted, thereby deploying the filter in the distal internal carotid artery. The filter allows distal blood flow while serving as an embolic filtration element within the artery lumen. Balloon angioplasty and stenting were then performed over the 0.014-inch filter wire.

After intervention, the retrieval catheter was advanced over the guidewire and through the stent, then further over the filter assembly. The retrieval is accomplished when the distal pod of the retrieval catheter contacts the proximal edge of the filter assembly, leading to the collapse of the nitinol expanders and the filtration element. The captured embolic particles are fully contained within the retrieval catheter. The entire device is then removed from the patient. A close-up view of the inside of the filter after carotid stenting showed that multiple embolic particles have been captured (Figure 3.3).

Commentary

Distal protection devices are being introduced into the carotid stenting procedure in order to capture atherosclerotic emboli and eliminate the risk of associated neurological embolic events. This case illustrates a simple technique in which the MedNova filter protection system is utilized during carotid stenting. The advantage of a distal protection filter in this case is the preservation of blood flow and the ability to perform angiography during the procedure. The large crossing profile of the current filters renders them difficult to be used in severe lesions and tortuous vessel anatomy. Additional maneuvers such as initial

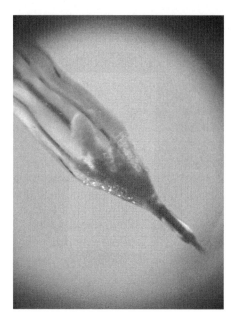

Figure 3.3 *Captured embolic debris is seen in a few patients who undergo carotid stenting with a distal protection system. A filter, from anther patient, contains embolic debris.*

dilatation using a small-profile balloon (e.g. 2.0 mm × 40 mm coronary balloon), positioning of a second coronary wire ('buddy wire'), and placement of the tip of the guiding sheath close to the lesion proximally, within the common carotid artery, may facilitate the crossing ability of the lesion with the filter system. The new generation over-the-wire filter system is overcoming this limitation with a lower profile and improved tractability.

CASE 4: CAROTID STENTING WITH FAILED DISTAL PROTECTION

Alan S Boulos, Andrew J Ringer,
Demetrius K Lopes, Lee R Guterman,
L Nelson Hopkins

Background

A 68-year-old man had previously undergone a right carotid endarterectomy for asymptomatic carotid stenosis, as well as an angioplasty of his left renal artery for renal stenosis. More recently, the patient developed angina pectoris with severe three-vessel stenosis on coronary angiography. After being referred for

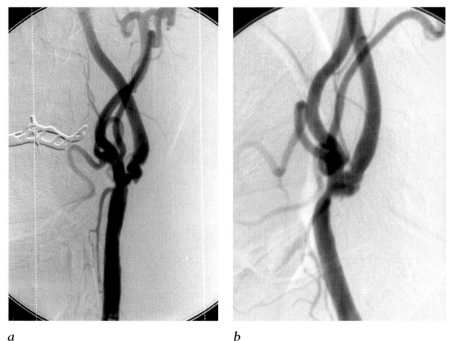

a   b

Figure 4.1 (a) Anteroposterior angiogram of the left common carotid artery (ICA) shows severe left internal carotid artery stenosis in an asymptomatic 68-year-old man. He was referred for carotid stenting as a result of his severe coronary artery disease. (b) Lateral view shows acute angulation of the ICA origin from the common carotid artery. (a, b) The external carotid origin was straight.

coronary artery bypass grafting, he was evaluated with carotid Doppler studies that demonstrated a left internal carotid artery (ICA) stenosis. Subsequent angiography confirmed the left ICA stenosis (Figure 4.1).

As a result of the requirement for coronary revascularization, he was considered to be at high risk for carotid endarterectomy and was referred for carotid stenting. As a high-risk coronary patient, he was also considered a candidate for participation in a clinical trial investigating the use of a carotid distal protection device. The protection device is a filter device, mounted on a guidewire. It is delivered in a constrained configuration within a delivery catheter and expands after satisfactory positioning upon removal of the delivery catheter. A soft, shapable extension of the wire leads the filter device to permit navigation of the carotid bifurcation.

Procedure

The procedure was performed under local anesthesia via the right transfemoral artery approach. After securing femoral access, heparin was administered to achieve an activating coagulation time of >300 s. Using a sheath and a Simmons two-curve catheter, we accessed the left common carotid artery. An exchange length super-stiff wire was positioned to place a 7 Fr guide sheath within the midcervical left common carotid artery.

We attempted to place the distal protection device across the ICA lesion. However, the origin of the ICA was quite angulated, and even though the filter wire would enter the ICA, the device would not track behind the wire – rather it prolapsed the wire into the external carotid artery (Figure 4.2). Multiple

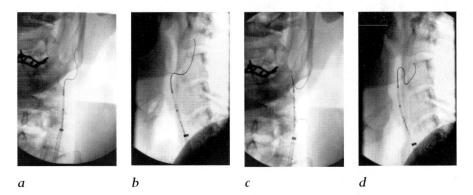

a   b   c   d

Figure 4.2 *(a) Anteroposterior and (b) lateral radiographs obtained during attempted positioning of a distal protection device. As the device first exits the guide sheath, the wire is directed into the internal carotid artery. Note the acute angulation of the internal carotid artery origin, which is easily crossed with the distal soft portion of the guidewire. As the device is advanced, however, it enters the external carotid artery in a straight trajectory, folding the soft leading portion of the wire: (c) anteroposterior; (d) lateral. The device was ultimately removed and not used in the procedure.*

attempts to position the device were unsuccessful, despite reshaping of the filter wire tip. We considered using a second, stiff 0.018-inch 'buddy' wire to straighten the trajectory into the ICA, but were concerned about disrupting the carotid plaque without stent protection. We chose to abort the attempted use of the distal protection device.

The lesion was crossed with a 0.014-inch wire and pre-dilated with a 4 mm × 40 mm angioplasty balloon at nominal pressure for 15 s. Asymptomatic bradycardia occurred during angioplasty and was successfully reversed by administering 0.75 mg atropine. After removing the angioplasty balloon, we positioned a 6- to 8-mm tapered Nitinol stent (40 mm in length) across the lesion and confirmed stent position with angiography (Figure 4.3). After stent deployment, the residual stenosis was corrected with a 5 mm × 20 mm angioplasty balloon with an excellent angiographic result (Figure 4.4).

The patient experienced no neurological symptoms throughout the procedure. After overnight observation in the intensive care unit, he was discharged without neurological deficit or hemodynamic compromise. Two months later, at his most recent follow-up visit, he remained neurologically intact and had no complaints referable to his procedure.

Commentary

The benefit of cerebral protection devices is clear. Unprotected carotid angioplasty and stenting carries a 5–10% incidence of events that result in

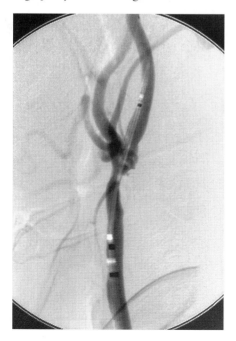

Figure 4.3 *Lateral angiogram of the left common carotid artery with a Nitinol stent in position before deployment. Note that the internal carotid artery origin has straightened when compared with the original angiogram in Figure 4.1.*

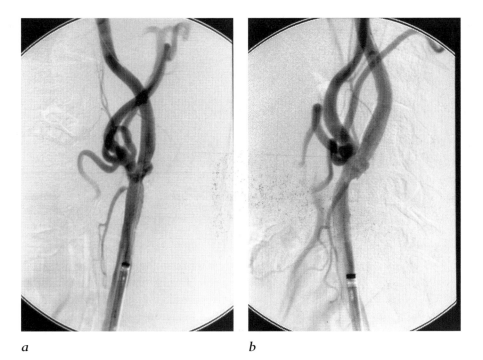

a   b

Figure 4.4 (a) Anteroposterior and (b) lateral angiograms of the left common carotid artery after stent deployment and post-stenting angioplasty. No significant stenosis remains and the patient remained neurologically intact.

neurological deficits. This rate is higher than in carotid endarterectomy. The most likely reason is that the microembolic load from carotid angioplasty and stenting is higher than with carotid endarterectomy. Angioplasty and stenting, however, result in less ischemia from hypoperfusion than endarterectomy. Therefore, if carotid angioplasty and stenting can be performed with a decreased embolic load, fewer neurological events will occur. Cerebral protection devices reduce this embolic load via three different potential techniques.

One method is distal internal carotid balloon occlusion during angioplasty and stenting. The disadvantages of this technique include potential ischemia from reduction of flow similar to that in endarterectomy, inability to perform angiography during balloon inflation, and risk of dissection or intimal injury of the ICA from balloon inflations. 'Dirty' blood is aspirated or allowed to exit the external carotid artery during balloon inflation. Potential emboli through the external carotid artery and into retinal or intracranial anastomoses may explain why some patients still experience ischemic events.

A second method involves inflating a balloon in the common carotid artery and aspirating blood during carotid angioplasty and stenting. The advantage of this technique is that the lesion is never crossed without protection already being instituted. A modification of this technique by Parodi adds an external carotid

17

balloon inflation to prevent emboli from going into the external carotid artery, and allows the ICA to be more effectively aspirated through an artificial fistula to the contralateral femoral vein. The disadvantages of this technique include cessation of anterograde flow during stenting and angioplasty, as well as creation of an arteriovenous fistula that could siphon flow from normal collateral paths in the brain. Other disadvantages include potential risk from embolic debris that has not been completely aspirated and removed.

Both occlusion techniques add considerable time and complexity to the procedure. The third technique is a filter device. Once the filter is in place, carotid angioplasty and stenting may proceed. The main advantage of this approach is maintenance of flow during the procedure. The disadvantages include potential generation of emboli from a large or stiff crossing device, possible loss of some particles smaller than the 100–150 μm filter pores, and intimal damage from a fully deployed filter.

This case demonstrates failure to deploy a filter-type distal protection device. The reason for failure was not the profile of the crossing device but rather the stiffness of the enclosed filter. The soft wire tip could easily be advanced into the ICA, but the stiffer encased filter would not follow this tip. The ICA was tortuous and exited the bifurcation at an acute angle, resulting in the filter preferentially taking the straighter external carotid route. The major change in stiffness between the ensheathed filter and the distal wire creates a hinge point that impedes successful crossing of angulated arteries, especially those with tight origin stenoses. One possible solution would have been to straighten the ICA by crossing it with a stiff microwire (0.014 or 0.018 inch). This 'buddy' wire technique may have straightened the ICA sufficiently to allow the filter to reach the distal side. This straightening technique, however, poses a small risk of carotid plaque dissection and embolization.

There appears to be a 5–10% risk of failure to deploy filters or distal balloons successfully. If deployment is successful, the filter is left in place throughout the procedure. Most filters must be placed in a straight arterial segment to optimize wall apposition and embolic capture. Enlargement of the artery during systole or after angioplasty, as well as recapture of the device, exposes the debris in the filter to the anterograde blood flow which may dislodge and release captured embolic debris. Therefore, the filters must be sized exactly and extreme care must be exercised to achieve optimum capture efficiency.

Two publications have demonstrated the utility of protection devices. Theron et al[10] used a distal occlusion balloon in 158 carotid angioplasty and stenting procedures with a perioperative neurological event rate of 1%. Parodi et al[9] used all three types of devices with a perioperative neurological event rate of 0% with each of the three devices. Cerebral protection devices have a role in carotid artery stenting, but which type of device will prove most effective is not clear. There are still some limitations of the current armamentarium and improvements could be made.

References

1. Diethrich EB, Ndiaye M, Reid DB, Stenting in the carotid artery: initial experience in 110 patients. *J Endovasc Surg* 1996;**3**:42–62.

2. Jordan WD, Voellinger DC, Fisher WS et al, A comparison of carotid angioplasty with stenting versus endarterectomy with regional anesthesia. *J Vasc Surg* 1998;**28**:397–403.

3. Mathur A, Roubin GS, Iyer SS et al, Predictors of stroke complicating carotid artery stenting. *Circulation* 1998;**97**:1239–45.

4. Yadav JS, Roubin GS, Iyer S et al: Elective stenting of the extracranial carotid arteries *Circulation* 1997;**95**:376-81.

5. Coggia M, Goeau-Brissonniere O, Duval JL et al, Embolic risk of the different stages of carotid bifurcation balloon angioplasty: an experimental study. *J Vasc Surg* 2000;**31**:550–7.

6. Crawley F, Clifton A, Buckenham T et al, Comparison of hemodynamic cerebral ischemia and microembolic signals during carotid endarterectomy and carotid angioplasty. *Stroke* 1997;**28**:2460–4.

7. Crawley F, Stygall J, Lunn S et al, Comparison of microembolism detected by transcranial Doppler and neuropsychological sequelae of carotid surgery and percutaneous transluminal angioplasty. *Stroke* 2000;**31**:1329–34.

8. Ohki T, Marin ML, Lyon RT et al, Ex vivo human carotid artery bifurcation stenting: correlation of lesion characteristics with embolic potential. *J Vasc Surg* 1998;27:463–71.

9. Parodi JC, La Mura R, Ferreira LM et al, Initial evaluation of carotid angioplasty and stenting with three different cerebral protection devices. *J Vasc Surg* 2000;**32**:1127–36.

10. Theron JG, Paynelle GG, Coskun O et al, Carotid artery stenosis: treatment with protected balloon angioplasty and stent placement. *Radiology* 1996;**201**:627–36.

CASE 5: BILATERAL VERTEBRAL ARTERY STENT PLACEMENT

J Stephen Jenkins

Background

The patient is an 82-year-old woman who complained of symptoms of vertebrobasilar insufficiency over the past 3 years. These spells include dizziness, and fainting. She was evaluated by a neurologist who ordered an aortic arch and four-vessel angiogram, which demonstrated severe bilateral vertebral artery stenoses. She was referred for intervention by the neurologist.

Procedure

A 8 Fr sheath was placed into the right common femoral artery and 10 000 IU heparin given. Attempts to cannulate the left vertebral artery selectively with a 6 Fr multipurpose catheter were unsuccessful. A 6 Fr JR-4 diagnostic catheter successfully cannulated the left vertebral and a 0.035-inch exchange-length Wholey (Malinckrodt, St Louis, MO) wire was advanced across the lesion, taking care to avoid the V4 segment. The diagnostic catheter was exchanged for a 8 Fr multipurpose coronary guiding catheter over the Wholey wire. A 4 mm × 2 cm Opta-5 balloon was used to predilate the lesion at 6 atm. Next, a Palmaz P154 (Cordis, Miami, FL) stent was mounted on the predilatation balloon and deployed at the lesion site at 12 atm. Angiography demonstrated moderate residual stenosis, so a 5 mm × 2 cm Opti-5 (Cordis) balloon was inflated to 14 atm within the stent (Figure 5.1).

Next a 6 Fr JR-4 diagnostic catheter was engaged in the ostium of the smaller right vertebral artery. Attempts to advance a 0.014-inch Sport guidewire (Guidant) were unsuccessful. A 8 Fr JR-4 guiding catheter was engaged and the 0.014-inch guidewire was able to cross the lesion. A 2 mm × 2 cm coronary angioplasty balloon was advanced across the lesion and inflated to 8 atm, with an excellent result (Figure 5.2). An excellent balloon result was obtained and the vessel was not stented due to the small vessel diameter. The patient did well after the procedure and was discharged home the next day. She has remained asymptomatic.

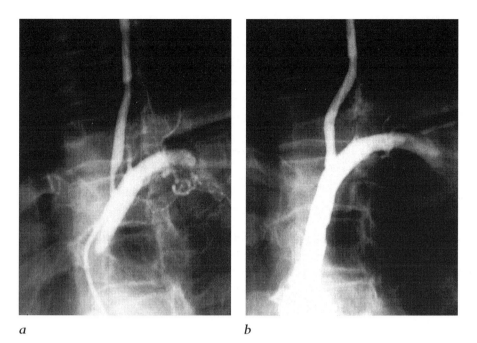

a   b

Figure 5.1. *(a) Seventy-five per cent stenosis of the dominant left vertebral artery. (b) Successful stent placement.*

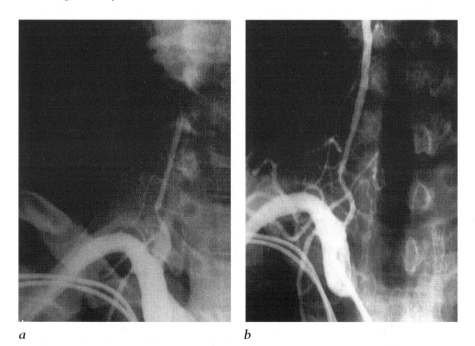

a   b

Figure 5.2. *(a) Subtotal occlusion of right vertebral artery (V2 segment). (b) Post-angioplasty result with brisk flow.*

Commentary

This case demonstrates the integration of both peripheral and coronary interventional equipment, which is often necessary to solve complex problems. The ability to take advantage of the availability of coronary equipment is a real advantage in successfully performing these procedures.

Case 6: Bilateral (Staged) Vertebral Artery Stent Placement

J Stephen Jenkins

Background

A 50-year-old man complained of vertebrobasilar insufficiency (VBI) manifested by dizziness and vertigo, which threatened his safety and stability at work. His symptoms were evaluated by a neurologist, who arranged an aortic arch and four-vessel cerebral angiogram: this demonstrated bilateral vertebral artery stenosis (Figures 6.1 and 6.2) As both vertebral arteries converge to form the

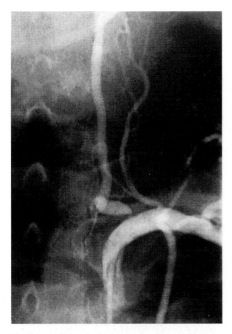

Figure 6.1 *This image demonstrates a high-grade ostial stenosis of the left vertebral artery. Approximately 2 cm distal to the ostium, the vessel makes a 90° turn cephalad. This gives an adequate window for angioplasty and stenting with a short stent.*

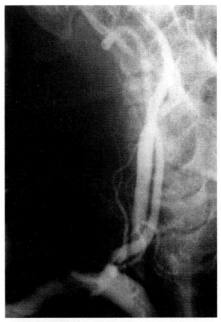

Figure 6.2 *This image represents a 95% stenosis of the right vertebral artery ostium. Transition to the bony canal of the V2 segment is smooth, lending this vessel more favorable anatomy for percutaneous angioplasty, with less risk of distal dissection.*

basilar artery, it was felt that the patient would benefit from revascularization of at least one of the vertebral arteries.

Procedure

Vascular access was obtained in the right common femoral artery with a 8 Fr sheath and 10 000 IU heparin were given. An additional 4000 IU heparin were given to maintain an activated clotting time (ACT) of over 300 s during the procedure. A diagnostic 6 Fr JR-4 catheter was used to cannulate the left subclavian artery and left vertebral artery ostium selectively. A 0.035-inch Wholey (Malinckrodt, St Louis, MO, USA) guidewire was then advanced into the V2 segment of the artery and the diagnostic catheter was exchanged for a 8 Fr JR-4 coronary guiding catheter. A 4 mm × 2 cm Opti-5 (Cordis, Miami, FL) angioplasty balloon was used to perform predilatation. A Palmaz P104 (Cordis) stent was mounted on a 5 mm × 2 cm Opti-5 balloon (Cordis) and deployed at the ostium of the left vertebral artery (Figure 6.3). Note that the short stent allowed the tortuous segment of this artery to remain unchanged.

After the procedure the patient was discharged on aspirin 325 mg/day, and clopidogrel (Plavix) 75 mg/day for 1 month. The patient's VBI symptoms improved, but only partially. He returned in 2 months requesting that the right vertebral artery be treated due to partial resolution of the VBI symptoms.

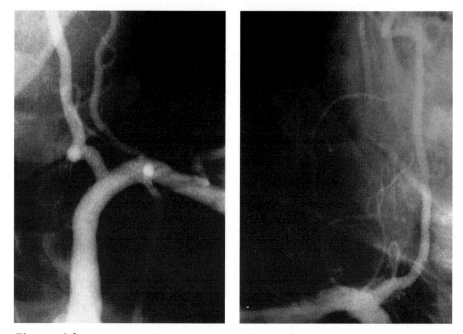

Figure 6.3 Angiography of the final result of the left vertebral stent.

Figure 6.4 Angiography of the final result in the right vertebral artery.

Vascular access was obtained with a 8 Fr sheath and heparin given to maintain the ACT > 300 s. A 5 Fr Van Andle (Cook) catheter was used to cannulate the right vertebral artery ostium. The 0.035-inch Wholey guidewire was advanced into the V2 segment of the artery taking care not to traumatize the V4 segment with the wire. (Two important branches, the posterior inferior cerebellar artery [PICA] and anterior spinal perforators, arise from this segment and care should be taken to protect these small vessels from guidewire trauma.) The diagnostic catheter was exchanged for a 8 Fr multipurpose coronary guiding catheter. Pre-dilatation was performed with a 5 mm x 2 cm Opti-5 balloon. A Palmaz P104 stent was mounted on the balloon and deployed in the ostium of the right vertebral artery at 12 atm. The final result demonstrates a widely patent ostium with a step-down seen at the distal end of the stent (Figure 6.4).

The patient did very well with complete resolution of his VBI symptoms for 6 months after which his symptoms partially returned. Angiography demonstrated in-stent restenosis of the left vertebral artery (Figure 6.5). This was treated with balloon angioplasty with an excellent angiographic and clinical result (Figure 6.6).

Commentary

This patient demonstrated a need for bilateral vertebral artery flow to resolve his symptoms completely, and, interestingly, to resolve the partial return of his symptoms with unilateral restenosis of the left vertebral artery at 6 months. Of note, the basilar artery and the posterior inferior cerebellar arteries were normal. Theoretically, revascularization of one vertebral artery should provide

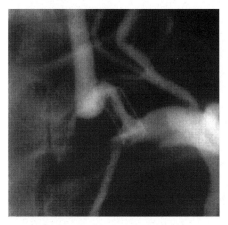

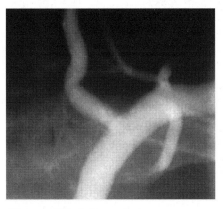

Figure 6.5 *This image of the left vertebral artery was taken 6 months after stent implantation. It demonstrates significant in-stent re-stenosis.*

Figure 6.6 *Left vertebral artery angiography after balloon angioplasty of in-stent re-stenosis.*

25

adequate flow to the posterior circulation, relieving VBI symptoms. Although it has been reported that one vertebral artery is adequate to prevent symptoms of VBI in humans, this was clearly not adequate to relieve symptoms in this patient.

References

1. Molnar RG, Naslund TC, Vertebral artery surgery. *Surg Clin North Am* 1998;**78**:901–13.

2. Berguer R, Long-term results of vertebral artery reconstruction. In: Yao JST, Pearce WH, eds, *Long Term Results in Vascular Surgery*, Norwalk, CT: Appleton & Lange, 1993:69.

3. Jenkins JS, White CJ, Ramee SR et al, Vertebral insufficiency: When to intervene and how? *Curr Intervent Cardiol Reports* 2000;**2**:91–4.

Case 7: Endovascular Treatment of Subclavian–Internal Mammary–Coronary Steal and Vertebral Preservation

Andrew C Eisenhauer, Joseph M Garasic

Background

A 47-year-old woman with left main coronary disease underwent coronary artery bypass grafting in which the left internal mammary artery (LIMA) was said to be 'small caliber' but was anastomosed to the left anterior descending artery; a saphenous vein graft (SVG) was placed to the second circumflex marginal branch. She was discharged without complications.

One week after discharge, she was admitted to another hospital with a non-Q-wave myocardial infarction. An urgent cardiac catheterization via the right femoral approach showed the left main lesion unchanged, a new lesion in the circumflex at the distal anastomosis site, the LIMA filled retrogradely and the SVG was closed.

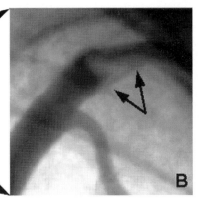
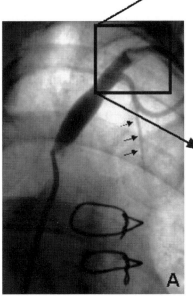

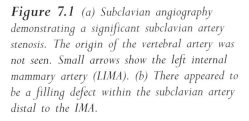

Figure 7.1 (a) Subclavian angiography demonstrating a significant subclavian artery stenosis. The origin of the vertebral artery was not seen. Small arrows show the left internal mammary artery (LIMA). (b) There appeared to be a filling defect within the subclavian artery distal to the IMA.

Subclavian angiography demonstrated a significant subclavian artery stenosis (Figure 7.1a). The origin of the vertebral artery was not seen. There appeared to be a filling defect within the subclavian artery distal to the LIMA (Figure 7.1b) The patient was placed on anticoagulant therapy and referred for treatment of the subclavian stenosis.

On arrival, additional detailed questioning revealed that the patient had noted left upper extremity cramping and soreness with use and elevation of the left extremity. In particular she noted pain and arm fatigue using a hair dryer and combing her hair. These arm symptoms had begun well before her coronary bypass procedure.

Procedure

We questioned whether the subclavian artery filling defects represented the inflow of non-opacified blood via collaterals and not thrombus. Subclavian angiography revealed a severe left subclavian stenosis involving the origin of the vertebral artery (Figure 7.2a). The small arrow indicates the thyrocervical trunk

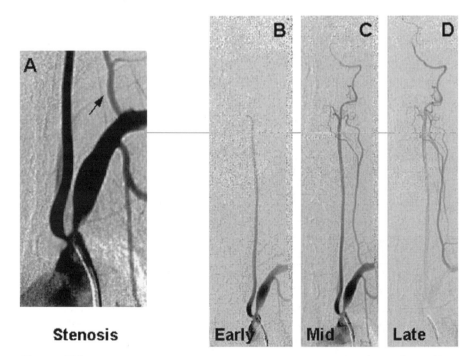

Figure 7.2 (a) Subclavian angiography revealed a severe proximal left subclavian stenosis involving the origin of the vertebral artery. The small arrow indicates the thyrocervical trunk and confirms that the 'filling defect' seen in Figure 7.1 was the inflow of non-opacified blood via this collateral vessel. (b–d) The left vertebral artery demonstrated delayed anterograde filling.

28

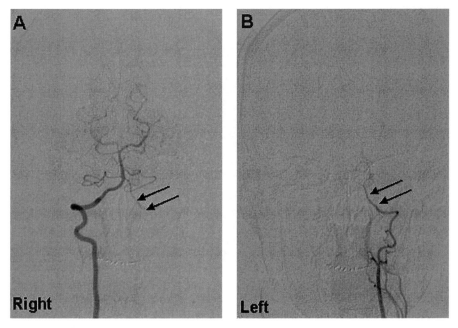

Figure 7.3 *(a) Selective angiography of the right vertebral artery, revealed that it supplied the basilar artery and retrogradely filled a portion of the left vertebral artery (arrows). (b) There was little or no contribution to the basilar by the left vertebral.*

and confirms that the 'filling defect' seen in Figure 7.1 was the inflow of non-opacified blood via this collateral vessel.

The left vertebral artery demonstrated delayed anterograde filling (Figure 7.2 b–d). Selective angiography of the right vertebral artery (Figure 7.3), revealed that it supplied the basilar artery. As the left vertebral artery was involved in the subclavian stenosis, it did not contribute to 'subclavian steal', but stenting of the subclavian artery could further compromise flow in the left vertebral artery. We believed it necessary (1) to relieve the subclavian stenosis to treat subclavian-IMA steal and arm claudication, and (2) to preserve and augment the perfusion of the basilar artery through the left vertebral artery. We did not plan to address the stenosis of the circumflex system at this time.

After diagnostic angiography, a 7 Fr long sheath was selected and positioned at the left subclavian origin. The subclavian was carefully pre-dilated with an undersized balloon, and a Guidant 28-mm Megalink stent mounted on a 7-mm balloon was carefully positioned covering the stenosis and slightly extending into the aorta (Figure 7.4a). The stent was deployed at low pressure with immediate angiography, showing incomplete stent expansion (large arrow) but continued, although compromised, patency of the origin of the vertebral artery (small arrow) (Figure 7.4b). The vertebral artery was quickly crossed with an 0.014-inch Graphix guidewire and a 4 mm × 15 mm Quantum Ranger balloon was advanced and a final 'kissing' inflation made at higher pressure (Figure 7.4c).

29

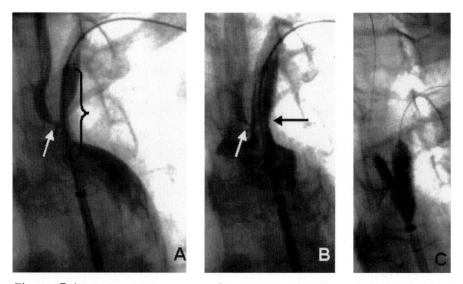

Figure 7.4 *(a) The subclavian was carefully pre-dilated with an undersized balloon and a Guidant 28-mm Megalink stent mounted on a 7-mm balloon was carefully positioned covering the stenosis and slightly extending into the aorta. (b) The stent was deployed at low pressure with immediate angiography, showing incomplete stent expansion (black arrow) but continued, although compromised, patency of the origin of the vertebral (white arrow). (c) The vertebral artery was quickly crossed with an 0.014-inch Graphix guidewire and a 4 mm × 15 mm Quantum Ranger balloon was advanced and a final 'kissing' inflation made at higher pressure.*

Final angiography (Figure 7.5a) shows resolution of both lesions (the origin of the vertebral did not require a stent) and more vigorous contribution to the basilar artery by the left vertebral artery (Figure 7.5 b–d). Figure 7.6 compares the left (a) and right (b) anterior oblique views, demonstrating anterograde flow in the vertebral artery (single arrow), thyrocervical trunk (double arrows) and IMAs (triple arrows).

The vascular sheath was removed and the arterial puncture closed with a Perclose device. The patient was ambulatory and did not have angina, dizziness, vertigo or other symptoms. As she lived far from our institution, a low level exercise test was performed before discharge. She exercised for 9 min on a modified Bruce protocol and reported no chest or arm pain, had no arrhythmias and no ECG changes of ischemia. She was able to use a hair dryer and comb her hair without discomfort. At 6-month follow-up she was free of angina and arm claudication, and had no vertebrobasilar symptoms.

Commentary

The classic subclavian steal syndrome arises because of reversal of flow in the vertebral artery as blood is shunted into the brachial circulation. In most patients,

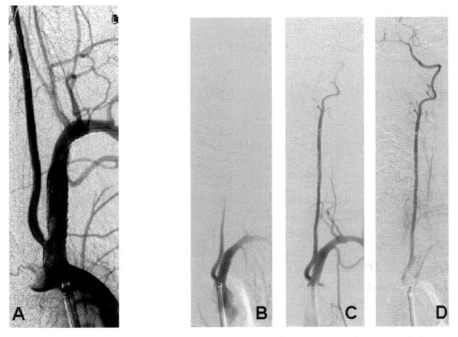

Figure 7.5 *(a) Final angiography shows resolution of both lesions (the origin of the vertebral did not require a stent). (b–d) More vigorous contribution to the basilar artery by the left vertebral.*

these symptoms are related to vertebrobasilar insufficiency and include dizziness, syncope and vertigo.[1] Upper extremity ischemic symptoms may occur as a result of ipsilateral claudication related to arm exercise or embolization to the digits.[2] In the coronary–subclavian steal syndrome, there is a proximal subclavian stenosis causing reversal of flow in the LIMA and ischemia of the myocardium.[3]

This case illustrates several important features of brachiocephalic and vertebral intervention. First, it is important to be aware of the potential for subclavian

Figure 7.6 *Compares (a) the left and (b) the right anterior oblique views demonstrating anterograde flow in the vertebral (single arrow), thyrocervical trunk (double arrows) and internal mammary arteries (triple arrows).*

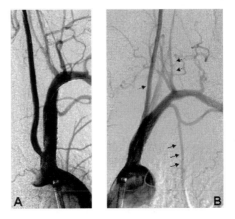

disease to compromise the results of surgical coronary revascularization, which could have been detected preoperatively by simply measuring the blood pressure in both arms. Second, the symptoms of arm claudication are often overlooked or misinterpreted as angina in patients with coronary disease. Third, the relationship of the subclavian stenosis to the IMA, the vertebral artery and other collateral vessels is important to document and understand before performing any intervention. Finally, the full range of interventional techniques and equipment, both peripheral and coronary, should be brought to bear on these complex problems to optimize therapeutic outcomes.

Subclavian artery lesions are usually pre-dilated with a slightly undersized balloon and then stented with a balloon-expandable stent sized 1:1 with the reference diameter. Stent placement must be precise. It is important when treating aorto-ostial lesions to ensure that the stent protrudes slightly (1–2 mm) into the aorta to ensure good coverage of the ostium. Most operators favor balloon-expandable stents at aorto-ostial locations, with self-expanding stents reserved for long segment disease or situations where more flexibility is needed.

Only indirect comparisons of endovascular and surgical approaches are available; no randomized trials have been performed. The initial technical success of surgery is high (mean 96%). The major complication of stroke occurs in about 3% and death in 2% of patients. Risk factors associated with complications suggested that open-chest procedures are associated with a higher mortality and morbidity than those for extrathoracic bypasses.[4–7]

Endovascular procedural success is equivalent to surgical approaches with fewer complications. Al-Mubarak et al[8] reported no strokes in their series of 38 patients, and strokes occurred in only 0.9% of subclavian procedures described by Henry and colleagues.[9] In addition, treatment failures occurred only in totally occluded arteries. Primary patency ranged from 94% at 20 months to 75% at 8 years, with overall patency of 100% at 20 months to 90% at 8 years.

Percutaneous endovascular revascularization of subclavian lesions with stenting has become the treatment of choice because it is less invasive with fewer complications. Contemporary reports have presented initial success and mid-term patency rates similar to those of surgery.[10] In addition, stenting may reduce the long-term risk of embolization and achieve anatomically and physiologically superior results, and is minimally invasive. As in all endovascular treatment, a careful appreciation of the anatomy, physiology and potential complications is critical to the development of a therapeutic plan and its successful implementation.[11]

References

1. Fields WS, Lemak NA, Joint study of extracranial arterial occlusion. Subclavian steal – a review of 168 cases. *JAMA* 1972;**222**:1139–43.

2. Bryan AJ, Hicks E, Lewis MH, Unilateral digital ischemia secondary to embolization from subclavian atheroma. *Ann R Coll Surg Engl* 1989;**71**:140–2.

3. Breall JA, Kim D, Baim DS, Skillman JJ, Grossman W, Coronary-subclavian steal: an unusual cause of angina pectoris after successful internal mammary–coronary artery bypass grafting. *Cathet Cardiovasc Diagn* 1991;**24**:274–6.

4. Berguer R, Morasch MD, Kline RA, Transthoracic repair of innominate and common carotid artery disease: Immediate and long-term outcome for 100 consecutive surgical reocnstructions. *J Vasc Surg* 1998;**27**:34–42.

5. Taha AA, Vahl AC, DeJong SC et al, Reconstruction of the supra-aortic trunks. *Eur J Surg* 1999;**165**:314–18.

6. Azakie A, McElhinney DB, Higashima R et al, Inominate artery reconstruction: over three decades of experience. *Ann Surg* 1998:**228**:402–10.

7. Mingoli A, Sapienza P, Feldhaus RJ et al, Long-term results and outcomes of crossover axilloaxillary bypass grafting: A 24-year experience. *J Vasc Surg* 1999;**29**:894–901.

8. Al-Mubarak N, Liu MW, Dean LS et al, Immediate and late outcomes of subclavian artery stenting. *Cathet Cardiovasc Intervent* 1999;**46**:169–72.

9. Henry M, Amor M, Henry I, Ethevenot G, Tzvetanov K, Chati Z, Percutaneous transluminal angioplasty of the subclavian arteries. *J Endovasc Surg* 1999;**6**:33–41.

10. Hadjipetrou P, Cox S, Piemonte T, Eisenhauer A, Percutaneous revascularization of atherosclerotic obstruction of aortic arch vessels [see comments]. *J Am Coll Cardiol* 1999;**33**:1238–45.

11. Eisenhauer A, Subclavian and innominate revascularization: surgical therapy versus catheter-based intervention. *Curr Intervent Cardiol Reports* 2000;**2**:101–10.

CASE 8: SUBCLAVIAN ARTERY INTERVENTION

Gustav R Eles, Simon Chough, Mark Wholey

Background

A 68-year-old woman presented with exertional angina. She had undergone coronary artery bypass surgery 6 years earlier, including a left internal mammary artery graft to the left anterior descending artery. A radionuclide stress examination demonstrated reversible anteroseptal ischemia. Her physical examination was remarkable because the left arm systolic blood pressure was 80 mmHg less than the right arm. Doppler ultrasound studies were consistent with left-sided subclavian steal syndrome.

Procedure

Diagnostic angiography was performed with a 6 Fr diagnostic JR-4 catheter from the common femoral artery. A severe stenosis of the proximal left subclavian artery was confirmed (Figure 8.1). Contrast injection into the native left coronary system demonstrated prominent retrograde filling of the internal mammary graft, suggesting subclavian steal.

A 8 Fr sheath was inserted over a wire. The patient was heparinized. The 6 Fr JR-4 diagnostic catheter was re-engaged in the ostium of the left subclavian artery. The lesion was crossed with an exchange-length 0.035-inch Wholey wire (Mallinkrodt, St Louis, MO, USA). The diagnostic catheter was changed for a 8

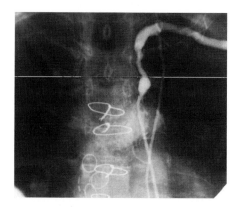

Figure 8.1 *Angiography with a 6 Fr JR-4 diagnostic catheter, demonstrating severe proximal left subclavian artery stenosis.*

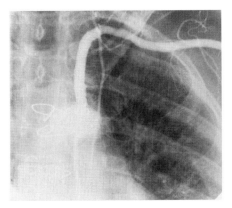

Figure 8.2 *Post-stent angiography with resolution of subclavian artery stenosis.*

Fr multipurpose guide catheter (Cordis, Miami, FL). A PowerFlex (Cordis) 6 mm × 40 mm balloon catheter was passed into the stenosis. Balloon angioplasty was performed to a maximum pressure of 8 atm. Repeat angiography demonstrated significant recoil within the lesion and it was decided to proceed with stent placement. A Palmaz P394M (Cordis) stent was deployed using the same angioplasty balloon. The maximum pressure applied was 12 atm. Repeat angiography demonstrated an excellent result (Figure 8.2). The exertional angina disappeared immediately after the procedure and the follow-up exercise perfusion imaging was normal.

Commentary

Coronary–subclavian steal has been recognized with increasing frequency as the use of the internal mammary artery as a bypass conduit has become popular. In the past, carotid–subclavian bypass was used to treat patients with symptomatic subclavian steal syndrome. As percutaneous intervention developed, reports of catheter-based treatment began to surface. Current technology greatly improves the likelihood of successful outcomes.

Patients with known coronary artery disease should be screened for peripheral vascular disease, as the two entities often coexist. Patients preparing to undergo coronary artery bypass grafting should be examined specifically for subclavian artery stenosis.

References

1. Marshall WG, Miller EC, Kouchoukos NT, The coronary-subclavian steal syndrome: report of a case and recommendations for prevention and management. *Ann Thorac Surg* 1988;**46**:93.

35

2. Olson CO, Dunton FR, Maggs PR, Lahey SJ, review of coronary-subclavian steal following internal mammary artery–coronary artery bypass surgery. *Ann Thorac Surg* 1988;**46**:675.

3. Meranze SG, McLean GK, Burke DR, Balloon dilatation of a subclavian artery stenosis proximal to an internal mammary-coronary artery bypass graft. *J Intervent Radiol* 1986;**1**:83.

4. Ishii K, Hirota Y, Kita Y et al, Coronary–subclavian steal corrected with percutaneous transluminal angioplasty. *J Cardiovasc Surg* 1991;**32**:275.

5. Soulen MC, Sullivan KL, Subclavian artery angioplasty proximal to a left internal mammary–coronary artery bypass graft. *Cardiovasc Intervent Radiol* 1991;**14**:355.

6. Levitt RG, Wholey MH, Jarmolowski CR, Subclavian artery angioplasty for treatment of upper extremity claudication, subclavian and coronary artery steal syndromes. *J Vasc Intervent Radiol* 1991;**2**:48.

Case 9: Left subclavian artery intervention: LIMA graft perfusion and arm claudication

James Hermiller

Background

A 64-year-old man, presented with progressive angina and left arm claudication. He had undergone bypass surgery, including a left internal mammary artery (LIMA) to the left anterior descending artery (LAD), 10 years before admission. Physical examination was notable because of a 40 mmHg systolic blood pressure gradient in the left arm. The patient underwent cardiac catheterization and was found to have patent grafts. Cervicocerebral arch and carotid angiography demonstrated widely patent great vessels, except for an 80% stenosis of the proximal left subclavian artery; the left vertebral artery arose directly from the aorta. He subsequently underwent percutaneous transluminal angioplasty (PTA) of the subclavian artery (Figure 9.1) with a 8 mm × 4 cm balloon to 8 atm. Post-PTA angiography (Figure 9.2) demonstrated a widely patent vessel with what was thought to be a stable dissection. Five days later he developed acute left arm ischemia. Radial and brachial pulses were absent; there was no evidence of distal embolization. Following initiation of intravenous heparin, weak pulses returned in the left upper extremity.

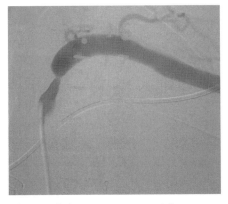

Figure 9.1 Pre-intervention left subclavian angiogram.

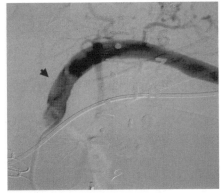

Figure 9.2 Angiogram after percutaneous transluminal angioplasty with arrow denoting dissection.

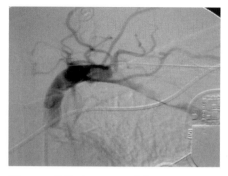

Figure 9.3 *Angiogram following subacute vessel closure 5 days after percutaneous transluminal angioplasty.*

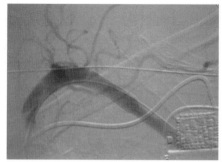

Figure 9.4 *Post-Wallstent placement distal to the internal mammary artery.*

He underwent repeat angiography (Figure 9.3) which demonstrated subclavian occlusion beyond the LIMA, extending to the axillary artery and resulting from a spiral dissection originating at the PTA site. A 4 Fr headhunter catheter was used to engage the artery, and a 0.035-inch TAD wire was used judiciously to cross the occlusion. A local infusion of tissue plasminogen activator (tPA) was given without improvement in the appearance of the vessel. A 9 Fr multipurpose guide was then exchanged for the infusion catheter and a 10-mm diameter self-expanding Wallstent (Boston Scientific Corp., Boston, MA, USA) was deployed distal to the LIMA. Figure 9.4 demonstrates that, after the self-expanding stent, the proximal dissection persisted. After deployment of a Palmaz (Cordis, Miami, FL) balloon-expandable stent proximally (dilated to 8 mm), there was no residual dissection, with preservation of the LIMA flow (Figure 9.5). Re-look angiography 6 months later for recurrent chest pain demonstrated widely patent stent sites.

Commentary

This patient's presentation was typical; his post-interventional course was unusual. A relatively uncommon and often unrecognized disorder, subclavian

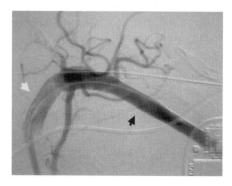

Figure 9.5 *Final angiogram after placement of a Palmaz stent (white arrow) proximal to the internal mammary artery (site of original stenosis) and Wallstent distally (black arrow).*

stenosis is present in 5% of those undergoing diagnostic heart catheterization before coronary artery bypass grafting (CABG).[1,2] It is much more common than disease of the innominate artery, and the left subclavian artery is affected five times more frequently than the right.[3] As in this case, atherosclerosis is the predominant etiology, although occasionally arteritis and radiation can be the cause. Patients may present with vertebrobasilar complaints resulting from subclavian steal, upper extremity claudication and/or angina in those with previous IMA grafting. Differential blood pressures and a history of peripheral vascular disease are independent predictors of subclavian disease.[4]

Percutaneous intervention is the preferred therapy. Femoral access is used except for total occlusions and a severely angulated geometry where a brachial approach is preferred. As in this case, the vessel is accessed with 4 Fr or 5 Fr diagnostic catheters and then crossed with a 0.035- or 0.018-inch wire. Subsequently the diagnostic catheter is exchanged for a 8 Fr multipurporse guide or 6 Fr long sheath. Pre-dilatation is routinely performed to enhance placement and ensure adequate stent expansion. Balloon-expandable stent systems are preferred because of their radial strength and precise positioning. As demonstrated in this case, self-expanding stents are used for severely angulated segments or lesions beyond the IMA, a location where external vessel compression is possible. Although PTA has been reported to be effective and safe, this case demonstrates an unusual complicaton–subacute vessel closure.[5] Other infrequent major complications include cerebrovascular accident/transient ischemic attack (<1%), distal emboli and side-branch closure. As a result of predictability, perceived lower re-stenosis rates (particularly in the treatment of total occlusions) and, in spite of a lack of randomized data, primary stenting has become the preferred treatment strategy for subclavian stenosis.[6–9]

References

1. Fields WS, Lemak NA, Joint study of extracranial arterial occlusion VII. subclavian steal: A review of 168 cases. *JAMA* 1972;**222**:1139–43.

2. English JL, Donovan DJ, Guidera SA, Carell ES, Angiographic prevalence and clinical predictors of left subclavian stenosis in patients undergoing diagnostic cardiac catheterization. *J Am Coll Cardiol* 1999;**33**:292A.

3. Phatouros CC, Higashida RT, Malek AM et al, Endovascular treatment of noncarotid extracranial cerebrovascular disease. *Neurosurg Clin N Am* 2000;**11**:331–50.

4. Wiliams SJ, Chronic upper extremity ischemia: Current concepts in management. *Surg Clin North Am* 1986;**66**:355–75.

5. Henry M, Amor M, Henry I, Tzvetanov K, Chati Z, Endoluminal treatment of sub-clavian occlusive diseases: Percutaneous angioplasty and stenting. *J Am Coll Cardiol* 1999;**33**;16A.

6. Hadjipetrou P, Cox S, Piemonte T, Eisenhauer A, Percutaneous revascularization of atherosclerotic obstruction of aortic arch vessels. *J Am Coll Cardiol* 1999;**33**:1238–45.

7. Ahuja R, Mishkel GJ, Kacich RL et al, Percutaneous interventions of subclavian artery occlusive disease. *J Am Coll Cardiol* 1999;**33**:16A.

8. Rodriguez-Lopez JA, Werner A, Martinez R, Torrulla LJ, Ray LI, Diethrich EB, Stenting for atherosclerotic occlusive disease of the subclavian artery. *Ann Vascular Surg* 1999;**13**:254–60.

9. White CJ, The times they are a-changin (editorial). *J Am Coll Cardiol* 1999;**33**:1246–7.

CASE 10 SUBCLAVIAN ARTERY STENT PLACEMENT

Suresh P Jain, Bahij Khuri

Background

A 54-year-old man presented with a 3-year history of right arm pain and dizziness associated with right arm movement. His past medical history was remarkable for having three coronary artery bypass grafts (CABGs), hypertension and hyperlipidemia. His clinical examination revealed bilateral carotid bruits with a weak radial pulse on the right side and a blood pressure difference of 40 mmHg between the two arms.

Procedure

Vascular access was obtained using the Seldinger technique via the right femoral artery. A 6 Fr sheath was introduced over a wire and 3000 U unfractionated heparin were administered. Selective four-vessel angiography was performed using JB 2 catheter (Cook Inc., Bloomington, IN, USA). Selective angiography of the right innominate artery was performed in 30° right anterior oblique and 20° caudal views which revealed a 90% occlusion of the right subclavian artery with an absence of antegrade flow in the right vertebral artery (Figure 10.1). The right and left carotid arteries showed a 50% stenosis of the right internal carotid artery and a 60% stenosis of the left internal carotid artery. The left vertebral artery revealed antegrade flow with retrograde filling of both the right vertebral and the right subclavian arteries. A diffuse 50–60% stenosis was noted in the terminal portion of the right vertebral artery (Figures 10.2 and 10.3).

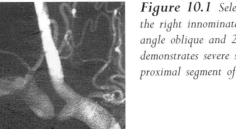

Figure 10.1 Selective angiography of the right innominate artery in 30° right angle oblique and 20° caudal views demonstrates severe stenosis (arrow) in the proximal segment of right subclavian artery.

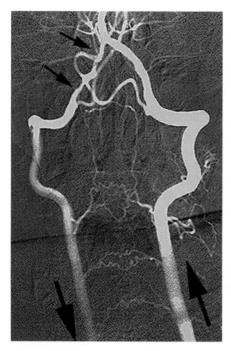

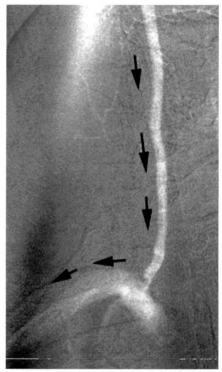

Figure 10.2 *Selective angiography of the left vertebral artery demonstrates anterograde flow (upward arrow) and retrograde flow in the right vertebral artery (downward arrow). Note the presence of diffuse 50–60% stenosis in the terminal part (small arrows) of the right vertebral artery.*

Figure 10.3 *Late phase angiogram of the left vertebral artery, demonstrating retrograde filling of the right vertebral artery and distal subclavian artery.*

An additional 3000 U unfractionated heparin were given and a 6 Fr right Judkins (JR-4) catheter was then used to canulate the ostium of the right subclavian artery. The lesion was crossed using a 180-cm long, stiff, angled Glidewire (Med-Tech, Boston Scientific Corporation, Watertown, MA). The JR-4 catheter was then advanced to the axillary artery and the Glidewire was exchanged for a 0.035-inch, 260-cm-long stiff Amplatz wire (Cook Inc). The Judkins catheter was then withdrawn over the wire and a 7 Fr 90-cm shuttle sheath (Cook Inc) was advanced to the ostium of the right subclavian artery. A simultaneous pressure gradient measurement across the lesion revealed a systolic gradient of 54 mmHg. The lesion was dilated with a 6 mm × 20 mm Opta-LP balloon (Cordis, Miami, FL) at 10 atm. The balloon was then advanced into the distal subclavian artery and the Amplatz wire was exchanged for 0.035-inch, 300-cm-long Wholey wire (Mallinckrodt Inc, St Louis, MO). An 18-mm Megalink stent (Guidant, Santa Clara, CA) was then deployed at the lesion site at 16 atm using a 7 mm × 20 mm Opta-LP balloon (Figure 10.4). Post-stent dilatation was performed using a 8 mm × 20 mm Opta-LP balloon at 18 atm. A simultaneous pressure gradient was recorded across the stent, which revealed a residual 10- to 12-mm gradient. A Viatrac balloon 135 cm long and 9 mm × 30 mm (Guidant, Santa Clara, CA) was used to dilate the stent at 10 atm.

Final angiography revealed excellent results with no residual stenosis and resumption of antegrade flow into the right vertebral artery (Figure 10.5). Repeat simultaneous pressure measurement across the stented lesion demonstrated no residual gradient. Physical examination revealed normal left radial and brachial pulses with equalization of blood pressure in both arms. The patient was discharged next day on clopidogrel 75 mg daily for 1 month and aspirin 325 mg/day indefinitely.

Commentary

The significance of this case is twofold: first, among patients with subclavian disease, the right subclavian artery is involved less frequently (20–30%) than the left subclavian artery. Second, the present case highlights the importance of coexisting extracranial and intracranial cerebrovascular disease in the genesis of subclavian steal syndrome. The presence of retrograde flow in the vertebral artery, either permanent or intermittent, does not determine neurologic symptoms. The severity of subclavian steal syndrome is proportional to the number of diseased cerebral arteries.

Surgical revascularization using transthoracic and extrathoracic approaches has been the standard treatment in symptomatic patients. In a recent review of surgical literature from 1966 to 1998 involving 2496 patients, Hadjipetrou et al[4] have reported an initial success rate of 95% with an overall complication rate of 16%. Major complications included stroke in 3% and death 2%. Other

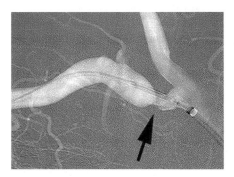

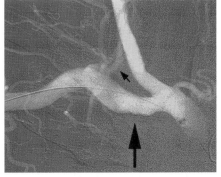

Figure 10.4 Angiogram showing positioning of Megalink stent across the stenosis for precise placement.

Figure 10.5 Post-stent angiogram demonstrates no residual stenosis and presence of antegrade flow in the right vertebral artery (small arrow).

complications included pneumothorax, myocardial infarction, phrenic nerve palsy, Horner's syndrome, delayed wound healing, wound infection, graft thrombosis, pleural effusion and chylothorax. A recurrence rate of 16% was noted over a mean follow-up of 51 months.

Bachman and co-workers[5] first described percutaneous transluminal angioplasty (PTA) of the subclavian artery in 1980. The major limitations of PTA include intimal dissection and high recurrence rate (range 20–54%). With the advent of endoluminal stenting, the technical success of catheter-based treatment has improved significantly. In a multicenter registry of subclavian and innominate artery stenting involving 258 patients, our group reported a procedural success rate of 98% with no peri-procedural stroke or death. Complications included peripheral emboli (1.1%), transient ischemic attack (TIA, 0.3%), access site thrombosis (0.3%), transient renal insufficiency (0.3%) and retroperitoneal bleed (0.7%).

Thus, compared with surgical treatment, endoluminal stenting of the subclavian artery provides equivalent or better initial success with lower complication and re-stenosis rates. It should be the treatment of choice for patients with subclavian and innominate artery stenosis. Endoluminal stenting offers significant advantages over standard surgical revascularization, which include no cervical or thoracic incision, no general anesthesia and a shorter hospital stay. It does not preclude further percutaneous interventions and surgical revascularization, if needed.

Clinical and technical points

1. Clinical manifestations of subclavian artery stenosis vary considerably. These include classic subclavian steal syndrome caused by posterior cerebral insufficiency, upper extremity ischemia resulting from limited flow to the arm as seen in the present case, coronary–subclavian steal syndrome caused by coronary flow reversal in a patient with a graft from the left internal mammary artery to the left anterior descending artery (LAD) and rarely plaque degeneration and distal embolization. A careful clinical examination and blood pressure measurement in both arms usually provide the diagnosis in suspected cases.

2. Aortic arch angiography in left anterior oblique projection provides information about the left subclavian artery and its distal course. However, this view does not lay out the bifurcation of the innominate artery into the right subclavian and right common carotid arteries. Innominate artery bifurcation is usually best seen in 20–30° right anterior oblique and 15–20° caudal view. This becomes important in cases of right subclavian ostial lesions, where precise placement of the stent without compromise of the ostium of the right common carotid artery is of paramount importance.

3. In patients presenting with subclavian steal syndrome, it is important to perform four-vessel angiography to rule out any extracranial or intracranial carotid disease or vertebral artery disease, which is quite frequently seen in patients with peripheral vascular disease. By affecting the collateral flow through the circle of Willis, these intracranial or extracranial lesions contribute to the genesis of the subclavian steal syndrome. In such cases, even successful treatment of the subclavian stenosis may not improve the underlying neurologic symptoms.

4. The left subclavian artery can be treated successfully using a femoral approach because of its direct take-off from the distal aortic arch. The right subclavian artery, because of its angulated take-off from the innominate artery, is usually best approached from the ipsilateral brachial artery. In the case of an ostial right subclavian artery lesion, placing a wire through the femoral access can protect the right common carotid artery. If needed, one can perform a 'kissing balloon' technique to protect the ostium of the right common carotid artery.

5. Total occlusions usually require a combined approach. Simultaneous angiography through both access sites allows pressure gradient measurements and better assessment of the lesion length. The short distance between the brachial artery and the subclavian artery occlusion enables better control of both the guidewire and the catheter, which assists in successfully crossing the lesion. It also allows usage of balloons with smaller lengths.

6. Stent delivery can be accomplished mostly using a 8 Fr multipurpose catheter or via a long 7 Fr shuttle sheath.

7. The selection of stent type and length depends on the size of the adjacent normal artery, lesion length and lesion location (ostial, proximal or distal beyond the vertebral artery). Balloon-expandable stents, such as the Palmaz or Corianthian stents (Johnson and Johnson, Warren, NJ), Megalink stent (Guidant Inc, Santa Clara, CA) and Bridge X3 stent (Medtronic AVE, Santa Rosa, CA), are best suited for ostial or proximal lesions. They can be delivered at a precise location more reliably than self-expanding stents. For distal subclavian artery lesions, a self-expanding stent (WallStent, SMART stent) is better suited because of its flexibility and ability to conform to the vessel tortuosity.

References

1. Fields WS, Lemak NA, Joint study of extracranial arterial occlusion: subclavian steal – a review of 168 cases. *JAMA* 1972;**222**:1139–43.

3. Hennerici M, Klemm C, Rautenberg W, The subclavian steal phenomenon: a common vascular disorder with rare neurologic deficits. *Neurology* 1988;**38**: 669–73.

3. Hutchinson EC, Yates PO, Carotid–vertebral stenosis. *Lancet* 1957;2–8.

4. Hadjipetrou P, Cox S, Piemonte T, Eisenhauer A, Percutaneous revascularization of atherosclerotic obstruction of aortic arch vessels. *J Am Coll Cardiol* 1999; 33:1238–45.

5. Bachman DM, Kim RM, Transluminal dilatation for subclavian steal syndrome. *AJR* 1980;**135**:995–6.

6. Herbrang A, Maskoic J, Tornac B, Percutaneous transluminal angioplasty of subclavian arteries: long term results in 52 patients. *AJR* 1991;**156**:1091–4.

7. Burke DR, Gordon RL, Mishkin J et al, Percutaneous transluminal angioplasty of subclavian artery. *Radiology* 1987;**164**:699–704.

8. Erbstein RA, Wholey MH, Smoot S, Subclavian artery steal syndrome: Treatment by percutaneous transluminal angioplasty. *AJR* 1988;291–4.

9. Farina C, Mingoli A, Schultz RD et al, Percutaneous transluminal angioplasty versus surgery for subclavian artery occlusive disease. *Am J Surg* 1989;**158**:511–14.

10. Jain SP, Ramee SR, Ansel GM et al, Endoluminal stenting of subclavian and innominate artery: Acute and long term results from a multicenter stent registry [abstract]. *Circulation* 1998;**98**:I–484.

CASE 11: OCCLUDED SUBCLAVIAN ARTERY INTERVENTION

Daniel T Lee, Robert D Safian

Background

This 55-year-old man was admitted for revascularization of an occluded left subclavian artery. He underwent coronary artery bypass graft (CABG) in January 2000, with a left internal mammary artery (LIMA) to the left anterior descending artery (LAD), saphenous vein graft (SVG) to the OM, and SVG to the right coronary artery (RCA). He developed recurrent angina 14 months after CABG and repeat angiography demonstrated total occlusion of the SVG to the OM, and high-grade stenosis of the proximal left subclavian artery. The stenotic proximal left subclavian artery was dissected and occluded during attempts to perform angiography. He underwent percutaneous transluminal coronary angioplasty (PTCA) stenting of the left circumflex artery but still had persistent angina, dyspnea, left arm claudication and vertebrobasilar insufficiency. A duplex ultrasound examination revealed a 40 mmHg pressure gradient between the left and right arm, reversed flow in the left vertebral artery consistent with subclavian and coronary artery steal, and normal carotid arteries bilaterally.

Procedure

As the left subclavian artery had a severe dissection and occlusion, retrograde (via the left brachial artery) and anterograde (via the right femoral artery) arterial access were obtained. Angiography demonstrated a long total occlusion from the ostium of the subclavian artery to the mid-subclavian artery, just proximal to the vertebral artery origin (Figures 11.1 and 11.2).

Despite multiple guidewires and catheters (0.035-inch straight and J-tipped glidewires, JR-4 and multipurpose catheters), we were unable to cross the lesion using a retrograde brachial approach. Ultimately, we successfully crossed the occlusion using an antegrade femoral approach with a 0.018-inch Gold glidewire (Boston Scientific/Vascular, Quincy, MA, USA) and an Ultrafuse-X catheter (Boston Scientific/Scimed, Maplegrove). This Gold glidewire was then exchanged for a 0.035-inch Magic Torque wire (Boston Scientific/Vascular) and balloon angioplasty was performed with a 7.0 mm × 20 mm Marshall balloon (Boston Scientific/Vascular). Despite satisfactory balloon expansion, there was no antegrade flow and persistent occlusion.

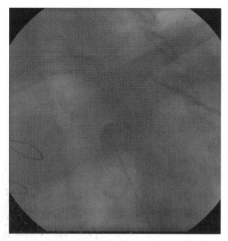

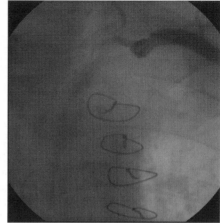

Figure 11.1 Antegrade angiogram showing proximal occlusion of the left subclavian artery.

Figure 11.2 Retrograde angiogram showing occlusion of the left subclavian artery just before the take-off of the vertebral artery.

For better definition of the anatomic landmarks for ideal stent position, angiography was performed using anterograde and retrograde approaches. Two Intratherapeutics Double Strut Stents (36 mm and 16 mm) (Intratherapeutics, St Paul, MN) were deployed using an 8 mm × 40 mm Marshall balloon and 8 Fr × 90 cm Arrow sheath (Arrow International, Reading, PA) as a stent delivery catheter (Figures 11.3 and 11.4). Final angiography revealed normal anterograde flow, no dissection or residual stenosis (Figure 11.5), wide patency of the LIMA and vertebral artery, and resolution of the translesional pressure gradient. The

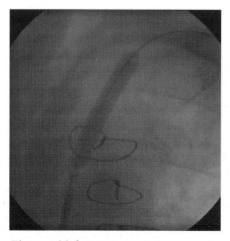

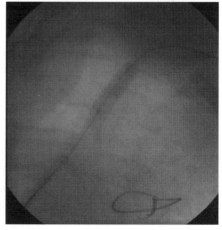

Figure 11.3 Initial stent placement in the proximal subclavian artery.

Figure 11.4 Second stent placement in continuity with the first stent to cover the lesion.

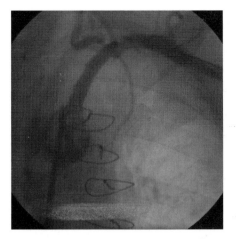

Figure 11.5 Final angiogram with widely patent vessels.

patient had immediate resolution of angina, dyspnea, left arm claudication and vertebrobasilar insufficiency.

Commentary

Clinical indications for subclavian or innominate artery revascularization include symptomatic subclavian steal syndrome, vertebrobasilar insufficiency, disabling arm claudication, and preservation of blood flow to the IMA or to an axillofemoral graft or dialysis conduit. This patient had subclavian stenosis and disabling arm claudication and coronary steal syndrome with vertebrobasilar insufficiency and angina. The incidence of brachiocephalic atherosclerosis is 20 times less frequent than atherosclerosis of the lower limb, and subclavian artery stenosis in patients undergoing CABG is reportedly 0.5–1.1%, which is probably seriously underestimated. The difference in arm blood pressure should be carefully assessed before CABG, and subclavian artery angiography should be performed at the time of coronary angiography if LIMA grafting is considered and if there are differential blood pressures between both arms.

The success rate for percutaneous revascularization of subclavian artery stenosis is 94–100%, but the success rate decreases to 75–80% for chronic total occlusion. Important technical considerations include the use of anterograde femoral access, retrograde brachial access or both, depending on the complexity and length of occlusion. Ideally, the stent should not protrude more than 1–2 mm into the aorta, and the distal edge of the stent should not compromise the integrity of the vertebral artery or IMA. We frequently rely on the 0.018-inch Gold glidewire, rather than the stiffer 0.035-inch glidewire, for initially crossing chronic total occlusions. The high technical success rate, low re-stenosis rate, minimal complications, short hospitalization, elimination of general anesthesia and low cost make percutaneous revascularization for subclavian artery occlusion preferable to surgical revascularization.

49

Case 12: Subclavian Steal Syndrome Secondary to Occlusion of the Left Subclavian Artery

Rajesh M Dave, Sumeet Sachdev,
Thomas M Shimshak

Background

A 69-year-old hypertensive woman presented with a 12-month history of progressive lightheadedness, dizziness, exertional left arm pain and intermittent paresthesiae of her left hand. She denied any history of chest pain, syncope, lower extremity claudication or visual symptoms.

She had blood pressures of 154/68 mmHg and 108/74 mmHg in the right and left arms, respectively. The carotid pulses were normal. A bruit was present over the left supra- and infraclavicular areas. The left axillary, brachial, radial and ulnar pulses were palpable but diminished compared with the right arm.

Arterial duplex imaging demonstrated a discrete lesion of the proximal left subclavian artery. In addition, there was reversal of flow through the left vertebral artery, consistent with subclavian steal syndrome. The carotid arteries were unremarkable and there was a mild, focal stenosis of the origin of the right vertebral artery.

Procedure

The patient was referred for angiography and percutaneous revascularization. Routine pre-medication was administered, including aspirin 325 mg/day. Selective visualization of the left subclavian artery was performed via the right femoral arterial approach using a 6 Fr left internal mammary artery (LIMA) diagnostic catheter. This demonstrated an occluded left subclavian artery at its origin from the aorta.

A second 5 Fr sheath was placed percutaneously into the left brachial artery and a bolus of 2500 U intra-arterial heparin was administered via the left brachial sheath. A 65-cm-long, 4 Fr, angled Terumo GlideCath (Boston Scientific Medi-Tech, Watertown, MA, USA) was then advanced through the brachial sheath over a 0.035-inch Wholey Hi-Torque Modified J guidewire (Mallinckrodt, St

Louis, MO), just proximal to the origin of the vertebral artery. Simultaneous contrast injections (10 ml iodixanol (Visipaque Nycomed, Inc, Princeton, NJ) were performed via the GlideCath and LIMA catheters (Figure 12.1). This demonstrated a fairly short occlusion which reconstituted proximal to the origin of the vertebral artery.

Based on the very proximal location of the lesion, we elected to recanalize the vessel from the left brachial arterial approach. A 0.035-inch angled Terumo glidewire (Boston Scientific Medi-Tech, Watertown, MA) was advanced to the distal limit of the occlusion through the 4 Fr angled GlideCath and then prolapsed through the occlusion without difficulty into the thoracic aorta. The GlideCath easily tracked over the wire through the occlusion into the aorta. A normal arterial pressure tracing was obtained to verify the correct location of the catheter. The catheter position was also confirmed by a manual contrast injection through the catheter.

The 0.035-inch Wholey wire was re-introduced through the GlideCath into the thoracic aorta. The GlideCath was exchanged for a 75-cm-long, 5.0 mm × 40 mm Marshall balloon catheter (Boston Scientific Medi-Tech) and overlapping inflations encompassing the ostium and occluded segment were performed (maximum inflation pressure of 8 atm).

It was our intention to stent (primary stenting) the recanalized left subclavian artery to optimize long-term patency. We exchanged the right femoral sheath for a 65-cm-long, 6 Fr, ArrowFlex sheath (Arrow, Reading, PA) and advanced this under fluoroscopic guidance over a 0.038-inch J wire to the arch of the aorta (Figure 12.2). A manual contrast injection through the femoral sheath was performed, demonstrating a patent vessel with significant residual disease. The left subclavian artery was engaged with the LIMA catheter, and a 0.035-inch Terumo glidewire was then advanced through the dilated left subclavian artery to the axillary artery. The LIMA catheter was then advanced over the 0.035-inch glidewire into the distal left subclavian artery. The Terumo glidewire was

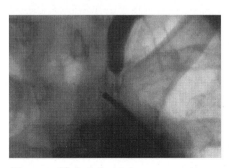

Figure 12.1 *Left subclavian arteriogram (anteroposterior projection).*

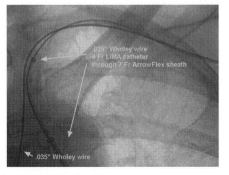

Figure 12.2 *Double-wire access of recanalized left subclavian artery (anteroposterior projection).*

51

exchanged for a 0.014-inch Hi-Torque Floppy II guidewire (Guidant Advanced Cardiovascular Systems, Temecula, CA) (300 cm) and the LIMA catheter was removed. The guidewire from the left brachial artery was also removed at this point. A 6.5 mm × 18 mm RX HercuLink (Guidant Advanced Cardiovascular Systems) stent was advanced through the femoral sheath which had been positioned just beyond the recanalized occluded segment. The sheath was withdrawn into the aorta and the stent was deployed at 10 atm (Figure 12.3). Final contrast injections demonstrated wide patency of the left subclavian artery and stent, brisk flow and a moderate ostial stenosis of the left vertebral artery which was not treated (Figure 12.4). An activated clotting time was obtained, intravenous protamine was administered and the arterial sheaths were withdrawn. The patient remained on combined aspirin 325 mg/day and clopidogrel 75 mg/day for 30 days.

Commentary

Occlusive disease of the subclavian artery has an incidence of 0.5–2% and is usually caused by atherosclerosis. The left subclavian artery is three to four times more commonly involved than the right. Clinical manifestations include exertional upper limb ischemia and/or symptoms of vertebrobasilar insufficiency (lightheadedness, dizziness, blurred vision, ataxia and/or syncope). Patients with prior coronary artery bypass surgery using the LIMA may present with subclavian–coronary steal syndrome and angina pectoris.

Left subclavian occlusive disease most commonly involves the ostium and/or proximal portion of the vessel. In general, percutaneous revascularization for ostial–proximal stenotic disease can be approached from the femoral access using long sheaths or guiding catheters. However, the brachial approach is useful for

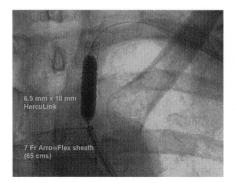

Figure 12.3 *Stent deployment at left subclavian artery ostium via the transfemoral approach.*

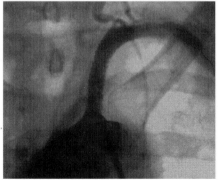

Figure 12.4 *Left subclavian arteriogram after angioplasty and stenting (anteroposterior projection).*

chronic total occlusions, defining the length of the occlusion and its relationship to the vertebral and mammary arteries, and providing maximum catheter support to cross the lesion. Intracerebral distal embolization during percutaneous intervention is felt to be reduced by delayed restoration of antegrade flow in the vertebral artery.[2]

Predicted procedural success rates for focal occlusive disease using balloon angioplasty and stenting are 92–97% with major complication rates at less than 1%. Success rates for chronic total occlusions have historically been in the 46–83% range. We have found the recanalization technique for chronic total occlusions used in this case to be extremely effective, with success rates of greater than 95%. Reported late re-stenosis rates have ranged from 6% to 19% with angioplasty compared with 10% for stenting. In general, balloon-expandable stents have been preferred for ostial-proximal lesions to maximize radial strength and for precise positioning. Caution should be exercised for angioplasty and/or stenting in close proximity to the verterbral and/or mammary arteries.

References

1. Perrault LP, Carrier M, Hudon G et al, Transluminal angioplasty of the subclavian artery in patients with internal mammary grafts. *Ann Thorac Surg* 1993;**56**:927–30.

2. Ringelstein EB, Zeumer H, Delayed reversal of vertebral artery blood flow following percutaneous transluminal angioplasty for subclavian steal syndrome. *Neuroradiology* 1984;**26**:189–98.

3. Becker GJ, Katzen BT, Dake MD, Noncoronary angioplasty. *Radiology* 1989;**170**:921–40.

4. Mathias KD, Luth I, Haarmann P, Percutaneous transluminal angioplasty of proximal subclavian artery occlusions. *Cardiovasc Intervent Radiol* 1993;**16**:214–18.

5. Motarjeme A, Percutaneous transluminal angioplasty of supra-aortic vessels. *J Endovascular Surg* 1996;**3**:171–81.

6. Al-Mubarak N, Liu MW, Dean LS et al, Immediate and late outcomes of subclavian artery stenting. *Catheter Cardiovasc Interv* 1999;**46**:169–72.

CASE 13: SUBCLAVIAN INTERVENTION FOR LIMA GRAFT PERFUSION

Patrick Whitlow, Christopher Bajzer

Background

A 73-year-old man presented with CCS class III crescendo angina. He had had a coronary artery bypass graft (CABG) 7 years ago including a left internal mammary artery (LIMA) graft to the left anterior descending artery (LAD) and two saphenous vein grafts (SVGs). He had also had bilateral carotid endarterectomies 8 years ago.

The patient denied upper extremity claudication or symptoms of vertebrobasilar insufficiency. Physical examination included no palpable pulses in the left arm. Diagnostic left heart catheterization demonstrated proximal occlusion of the native LAD, but a patent LIMA graft. However, there was high-grade stenosis with ulceration in the proximal left subclavian artery, jeopardizing the LAD territory (Figure 13.1).

Procedure

The femoral approach was chosen in this man because of ease of access (no palpable left brachial artery pulse) and the ability to use a large guiding catheter to accommodate high-profile balloons and stents while maintaining adequate opacification to place the stent precisely proximal to the origin of the vertebral artery and IMA. A 9 Fr guide and a balloon-expandable stent were chosen specifically to meet these challenges.

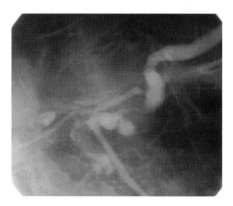

Figure 13.1 The severe proximal stenosis of the left subclavian artery with an ulcer crater just proximal to the most severe stenosis.

Figure 13.1 demonstrates the severe proximal stenosis of the left subclavian artery, with an ulcer crater just proximal to the most severe stenosis. The LIMA was identified distal to the stenosis. The left vertebral artery was not seen secondary to retrograde flow (as expected from a previous transcranial Doppler study).

The patient received heparin 50 U/kg, and the activated clotting time (ACT) was 250 s. The patient had been on chronic aspirin therapy, and ticlopidine 250 mg twice daily was begun 3 days before intervention. A 0.014-inch wire system was chosen for initial crossing in case pre-dilatation caused significant dissection into the mammary or vertebral artery. If branch compromise occurred, then the 0.014-inch wire could be used quickly to facilitate stent implantation in either of these branches using standard coronary equipment. Initially, a 0.014-inch/300-cm Shinobe Plus wire (Cordis, Inc., Miami, FL, USA) was used carefully to cross the complex ulceration. A 4.0 mm × 30 mm Ranger balloon (Boston Scientific, Maple Grove, MN) was then advanced past the stenosis and the Shinobe wire was exchanged for a 0.014-inch/300-cm Iron Man wire (Guidant Corp., Santa Clara, CA) to avoid potential injury as a result of migration of the distal tip of the hydrophilic wire. The balloon was then re-positioned and inflated to 10 atm for 2 min to try to stabilize any loosened plaque or thrombus (Figure 13.2). Angiography after angioplasty revealed brisk anterograde flow with mild intimal disruption and a residual 50% stenosis. There was no compromise of the origin of the LIMA or vertebral artery. The patient did experience ST segment elevation in the anterior leads, as well as chest discomfort with balloon inflation, which promptly resolved with balloon deflation. A 0.035-inch Tracker catheter (Boston Scientific/Target Therapeutics, Fremont, CA) was used to change the Iron Man wire to a 0.035-inch/300 cm Amplatz Super Stiff wire (Cook Inc., Bloomington, IN). A P294 stent (Cordis Corp., Miami, FL) was then hand crimped on a 7 mm × 30 mm ultrathin Diamond balloon (Boston Scientific, Quincy, MA) after removal of any lubricant coating with a sterile alcohol swab. The hand-crimped balloon-mounted stent was then advanced to the site of the stenosis, carefully positioned in several

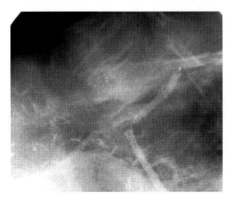

Figure 13.2 The coronary balloon was re-positioned and inflated to 10 atm for 2 min to try to stabilize any loosened plaque or thrombus.

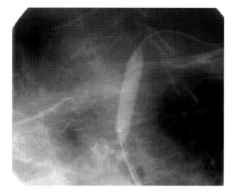

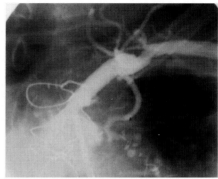

Figure 13.3 The hand-crimped, balloon-mounted stent was advanced to the site of the stenosis, carefully positioned in several angulated views and ultimately deployed at 14 atm.

Figure 13.4 Angiography after stent deployment revealed brisk anterograde flow with little residual stenosis and no intimal tear.

angulated views and ultimately deployed at 14 atm (Figure 13.3). Angiography after stent deployment revealed brisk anterograde flow with little residual stenosis and no intimal tear (Figure 13.4). There was continued normal flow down the mammary artery graft, and the vertebral artery was now clearly visualized with anterograde flow. A persistent small ulcer crater was visualized under the midportion of the stent. Strong radial and ulnar pulses were present.

The patient experienced no central nervous system (CNS) symptoms and no symptoms or signs of embolization to the left hand. The patient was subsequently discharged 1 day after the procedure with no complications and no angina.

Commentary

This case study illustrates one presentation of significant subclavian artery stenosis that would warrant revascularization. The approach was planned with careful consideration of potential complications at each stage of the procedure.

The choice of the femoral approach and the use of a 9 Fr guiding catheter facilitated the precise placement of a hand-crimped peripheral Palmaz stent without covering the vertebral or internal mammary origin. A self-expanding stent could be placed through a smaller guide catheter, but precise deployment is generally more difficult than with a balloon-expandable stent. The initial use of the optimally steerable and low-profile 0.014-inch wire allowed lesion crossing without embolization or dissection, and also allowed rapid rescue intervention to either the ostium of the vertebral artery or the ostium of the LIMA if these important vessels were compromised by angioplasty. The ability to

56

treat branch compromise quickly during subclavian artery intervention is critical for performing these cases safely. Respect for branch compromise was an important consideration in planning the entire interventional strategy for this man.

Potential embolic complications were also a concern with this bulky ulcerated plaque. Fortunately, no clinically relevant emboli occurred to the upper extremity, the heart or the CNS. The use of multiple wires was helpful in performing this case, allowing the operator to take advantage of the various unique strengths of the wires utilized – the sleek steerability of the 0.014-inch Shinobe plus, the soft tip and excellent support of the Iron Man, and the ultimate rail-like stability of the 0.035-inch Amplatz Super Stiff for tracking a rigid, large, profile stent.

Patients with successful subclavian stenting can be followed clinically with comparison of right and left arm blood pressures (and stress tests in the case of a patient with a patent internal mammary graft) as non-invasive indicators of re-stenosis. Probably because of the large lumina obtained with subclavian artery stenting, re-stenosis is an uncommon event. This particular patient has had no recurrence after 2 years of follow up.

References

1. Kumar K, Dorros G, Bates MC, Palmer L, Mathiak L, Dufek C, Primary stent deployment in occlusive subclavian artery disease. *Cathet Cardiovas Diag* 1995;**34**:281–5.

2. Sullivan TM, Gray BH, Bacharach JM et al, Angioplasty and primary stenting of the subclavian, innominate, and common carotid arteries in 83 patients. *J Vasc Surg* 1998;**28**:1059–65.

3. Henry M, Amor M, Henry I, Ethevenot G, Tzvetanov K, Chati Z, Percutaneous transluminal angioplasty of the subclavian arteries. J Endovas Surg 1999;**6**:33–41.

4. Al-Mubarak N, Liu MW, Dean LS, Al-Shaibi K, Chastain HD 2nd, Roubin GS, Immediate and late outcomes of subclavian artery stenting. *Cathet Cardiovas Interv* 1999; 46:169–72.

5. Rodriguez-Lopez JA, Werner A, Martinez R, Torruella LJ, Ray LI, Diethrich EB, Stenting for atherosclerotic occlusive disease of the subclavian artery. *Ann Vasc Surg* 1999;**13**:254–60.

Case 14: Innominate artery stent placement

Michael H Wholey

Background

A 76-year-old man presented with right arm claudication and dizziness. There was a discrepancy in the blood pressures of the two arms.

Procedure

Diagnostic angiography was performed from a common femoral approach with a 5 Fr pigtail catheter and an injection rate of 25 ml/s for 2 s (Figure 14.1) was performed. This revealed a calcified stenosis of 90% or more at the origin of the innominate artery.

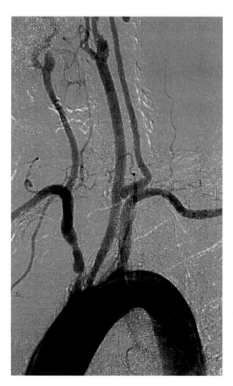

Figure 14.1 *Baseline aortogram demonstrating a tight lesion at the origin of the innominate artery.*

The patient returned 1 week later and a right brachial approach was chosen. Brachial artery access was selected because of the sharp angle that the innominate takes from the aorta. We prefer the antecubital brachial versus a middle or high brachial access, because of the difficulty in holding compression in someone who is muscular or has rolling arteries.

We used a micropuncture set (Cook Inc., Bloomington, IN, USA) to gain brachial access, then switched to a long 7 Fr flexible sheath. We crossed the lesion with a 0.035-inch glidewire (Terumo: Boston Scientific, Natick, MA) and predilated with a 4 mm × 2 cm balloon (Figure 14.2). The sheath was not advanced across the stenosis. A 28-mm-long balloon-expandable Megalink stent (ACS Guidant, Santa Clara, CA) mounted on a 7 mm × 4 cm Opta LP (Cordis, Miami, FL) was then deployed (Figure 14.3). Post-dilatation was not necessary based on angiographic findings (Figure 14.4). The patient had immediate improvement with equal blood pressures in both arms and absence of claudication.

Commentary

This is a straightforward procedure with expected success rates greater than 90% and with minimal risk in experienced hands, which can provide great benefit to the patient. The brachial approach, with smaller delivery systems, is an attractive alternative to the femoral approach. Symptoms may include vertebrobasilar insufficiency with ataxia, diploplia, syncope, vertigo, dizziness, nausea or vomiting and/or upper extremity ischemia with claudication atheroembolic digital ischemia.

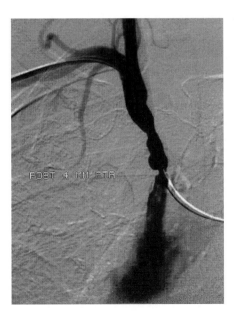

Figure 14.2 *Selective innominate angiogram after balloon predilatation.*

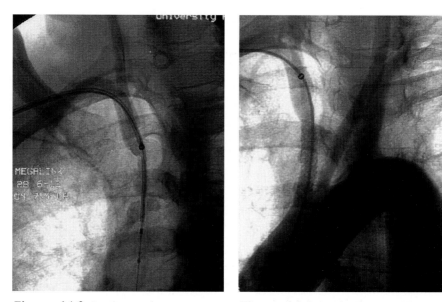

Figure 14.3 *Positioning the stent.*

Figure 14.4 *Final angiogram after stent deployment.*

The treatment of aorto-ostial innominate artery stenosis is similar to that of subclavian stenosis, except that care must be made not to compress the nearby left common carotid artery. There is consensus today that the treatment of choice in experienced hands for symptomatic aorto-ostial innominate stenosis is percutanoues intervention.

Recommended reading

Azzarone M, Cento M, Mazzei M et al, Symptomatic subtotal occlusion of the innominate artery treated with balloon angioplasty and stenting. *J Endovasc Ther* 2000;**7**:161–4.

Criado FJ, Wilson EP, Martin JA et al, Interventional techniques for treatment of disease in the brachiocephalic arteries (supra-aortic trunks). *J Invasive Cardiol* 2000;**12**:168–73.

Sullivan TM, Gray BH, Bacharach JM et al, Angioplasty and primary stenting of the subclavian, innominate, and common carotid arteries in 83 patients. *J Vasc Surg* 1998;**28**:1059–65.

Case 15: Angioplasty and Stenting of a Patient with Superior Vena Cava Syndrome

Debabrata Mukherjee, Bruce L Wilkoff,
Jay S Yadav

Background

A 45-year-old woman had a pacemaker implanted in 1994 and developed superior vena cava (SVC) syndrome in 1999. Despite medical treatment, she continued to have symptoms of facial and upper extremity edema, fatigue and sleep apnea. In September 2000, she developed a malfunctioning pacemaker lead, which required extraction and replacement. In view of severe symptoms of SVC syndrome and the need for pacemaker extraction and lead reimplantation, a decision was made to proceed with extraction of the lead system, angioplasty and stenting of the SVC, and reimplantation of the pacemaker lead.

Procedure

The patient was brought to the electrophysiology laboratory after informed consent was obtained. A right infraclavicular incision was made and the malfunctioning pacemaker and lead system easily removed. Diagnostic venograms showed complete occlusion of the right subclavian vein and severe stenosis of the SVC (Figure 15.1). A 8-Fr Mullins sheath system (Cook, Bloomington, IN, USA) was placed in the right cephalic vein and advanced to the subclavian vein. The lesion was crossed with a stiff, angled glidewire (Boston Scientific, Watertown, MA), placed inside a glide catheter (Boston Scientific, Watertown, MA) and the guidewire was advanced to the inferior vena cava (IVC). Balloon angioplasty was performed with a 8.0 mm × 40 mm Opta LP balloon catheter (Cordis, Miami, FL) at 8 atm for 60 s.

Subsequently, balloon angioplasty was performed with a 10 × 20 mm Opta LP balloon catheter, and then with a 12 mm × 40 mm Medi-Tech balloon catheter (Boston Scientific Corp.) at 9 atm for 60 s each. After balloon inflations there still remained severe stenosis (recoil) in the right subclavian vein (Figure 15.2). A 12 mm × 40 mm Nitinol self-expanding stent (SMART stent, Cordis, Miami,

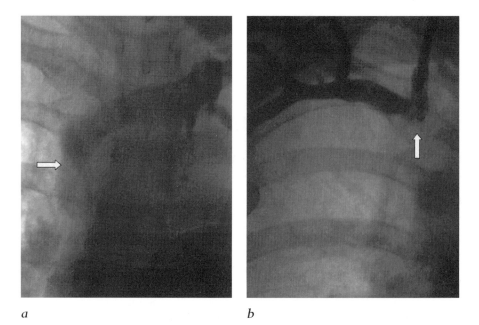

a   b

Figure 15.1 *Venogram from (a) the right cephalic and (b) the left brachial veins, demonstrating complete occlusion of the right subclavian vein and severe stenosis of the superior vena cava. The arrow in (b) shows occluded right subclavian vein and that in (a) demonstrates stenosis in the superior vena cava.*

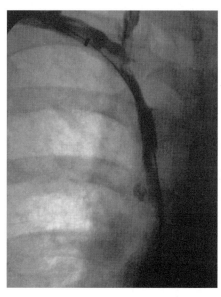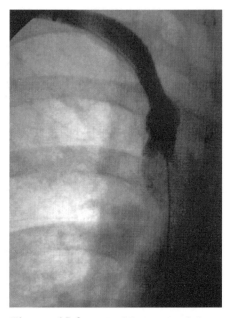

Figure 15.2 *Severe stenosis in the right subclavian vein after initial balloon inflation.*

Figure 15.3 *Successful stenting of the right subclavian vein with a 12 mm × 40 mm SMART stent.*

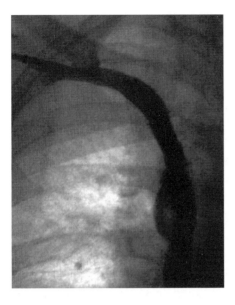

Figure 15.4 *Final angiography after implantation of a 14 mm × 20 mm SMART stent in the superior vena cava.*

FL) was deployed across the lesion in the right subclavian vein. The stent was post-dilated with the 12 mm × 40 mm Medi-Tech (Boston Scientific Corp.) balloon catheter at 10 atm for 55 s (Figure 15.3). The lesion in the SVC was dilated with the 12 mm × 40 mm Medi-Tech balloon catheter at 10 atm for 90 s. After this the Mullins sheath was advanced into the right atrium and gradients measured across the lesion in the SVC. There was a 8 mmHg residual gradient across the SVC lesion and a 14 mm × 20 mm SMART stent (Cordis) was advanced across the lesion in the SVC and deployed. The stent was post-dilated with the 12 mm × 40 mm Medi-Tech balloon at 12 atm. Gradients were remeasured across the SVC and the right subclavian vein, and there were no residual pressure gradients. Final angiography showed no residual lesions (Figure 15.4). A new pacemaker lead system was then placed through the stented right subclavian vein.

Commentary

We present a case of SVC syndrome after pacemaker placement in a young woman who was then successfully treated with percutaneous stenting. Obstruction of the SVC as a clinical entity affects approximately 15 000 people per year in the USA.[1] These patients can present either acutely or with a gradual worsening of symptoms, depending on development of collaterals.[2] Most cases of SVC syndrome now are related to malignancy, but occlusion of the SVC as a result of thrombosis or fibrosis caused by pacemaker leads is a recognized complication.[3,4] The reported frequency of this syndrome after pacemaker lead implantation has been variable, but several authors have now reported a frequency of 1 in 1000.[3] The precise pathogenesis has yet to be determined, but patients with two or more leads are three times more likely to develop complications.

If patients develop SVC syndrome after pacemaker lead implantation, they may require treatment either because of severe or refractory symptoms or because they may need SVC recanalization for lead replacement or implantation of additional transvenous catheters such as implantable defibrillators (ICDs), dialysis catheters or a Permacath for venous access.

Traditional management of SVC syndrome secondary to benign disease includes anticoagulation, elevation of the head and upper body, and cautious use of diuretics.[5] Despite these measures, approximately 40% of patients develop severe symptoms. Recently angioplasty and stenting have emerged as alternative treatment options for SVC syndrome.[1,5,6] The limitation of SVC angioplasty is the early re-stenosis caused by elastic recoil of the vein and venous compression from the mass or fibrosis that remains after the angioplasty.[4] Early re-stenosis has now been reported by several investigators, and stent placement would be the reasonable next step in endovascular therapy for SVC syndrome.

The case we presented has several interesting features, which include significant residual stenosis and a significant pressure gradient after balloon angioplasty, compatible with the severe fibrotic nature of the lesion. By using a Nitinol self-expanding stent with good radial strength, we were able to dilate the lesion adequately with resolution of the gradient. It is crucial to remove the leads first before stenting the vein, to preserve the future options of lead removal and to facilitate care in case re-stenosis develops. It is then optional to reimplant through the stents or from the other side. There were 170 000 pacemakers and 26 000 ICDs implanted in the USA in 1998.[7] As the number of patients with these devices increase, we are likely to see more patients with symptomatic SVC syndrome in the future. A number of patients will also probably be diagnosed when they present for lead extraction, lead replacement or insertion of additional transvenous catheters. Endovascular therapy with angioplasty and stenting appears to be a reasonable option in these individuals.

References

1. Yim CD, Sane SS, Bjarnason H, Superior vena cava stenting. *Radiol Clin North Am* 200;**38**:409–24.

2. Hochrein J, Bashore TM, O'Laughlin MP, Harrison JK, Percutaneous stenting of superior vena cava syndrome: a case report and review of the literature. *Am J Med* 1998;**104**:78–84.

3. Mazzetti H, Dussaut A, Tentori C, Dussaut E, Lazzari JO, Superior vena cava occlusion and/or syndrome related to pacemaker leads. *Am Heart J* 1993;**125**:831–7.

4. Marzo KP, Schwartz R, Glanz S, Early restenosis following percutaneous transluminal balloon angioplasty for the treatment of the superior vena caval syndrome due to pacemaker-induced stenosis. *Cathet Cardiovasc Diagn* 1995;**36**:128–31.

5. Kalman PG, Lindsay TF, Clarke K, Sniderman KW, Vanderburgh L, Management of upper extremity central venous obstruction using interventional radiology. *Ann Vasc Surg* 1998;**12**:202–6.

6. Schindler N, Vogelzang RI, Superior vena cava syndrome. Experience with endovascular stents and surgical therapy. *Surg Clin North Am* 1999;**79**:683–94.

7. American Heart Association, *Heart and Stroke Statistical Update*. Dallas TX: American Heart Association, 2001: 29–30.

CASE 16: SUBCLAVIAN VEIN THROMBOSIS

Aditya K Samal, Christopher J White,
Tyrone J Collins

Background

A 54-year-old patient with Hodgkin's lymphoma, in remission after radiotherapy,
developed left arm edema secondary to subclavian vein thrombosis. His totally
occluded subclavian artery was treated 6 weeks ago with local thrombolysis and
balloon angioplasty, with an excellent result. He was also started on wafarin
therapy to prevent re-thrombosis. Despite adequate anticoagulation, he now
returns with recurrent left arm swelling over the past 2 days.

Procedure

A 6 Fr sheath was placed in the right common femoral vein. Multiple
angiographic views of the left subclavian vein were obtained with a 6 Fr
multipurpose (MP) catheter (Figure 16.1). A 0.035-inch, exchange-length, angled
glidewire (Boston Scientific Corp., Watertown, MA, USA) was advanced across
the left subclavian vein occlusion, and the MP catheter was advanced over the
glidewire into the axillary vein. The glidewire was exchanged for a 0.035-inch

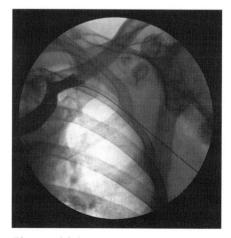

Figure 16.1 Occluded left subclavian
vein.

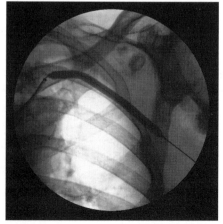

Figure 16.2 Inflated balloon across the
stenosis in the left subclavian vein.

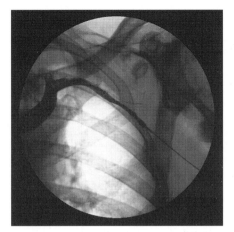

Figure 16.3 *Occluded left subclavian vein after balloon angioplasty.*

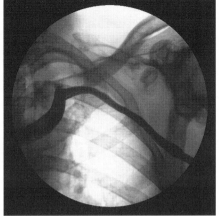

Figure 16.4 *Successful recanalization and excellent flow in the left subclavian vein after stent deployment.*

exchange-length, Wholey wire (Mallinckrodt, Inc., St Louis, MO), and the 6 Fr sheath and MP catheter were exchanged for a 90-cm-long, 7 Fr Shuttle sheath (Cook, Bloomington, IN). The subclavian vein was dilated with a 7 mm × 10 cm balloon up to a pressure of 8 atm (Figure 16.2). Angiography post-percutaneous transluminal angioplasty revealed significant recoil of the lesion (Figure 16.3). A 6 mm × 80 cm self-expanding SMART stent was advanced and deployed across the lesion. A post-stent deployment angiogram revealed residual stenosis proximal to the stent. A second 8 mm × 4 cm SMART stent was deployed proximal to the previously deployed stent. A post-stent deployment angiogram revealed successful recanalization and excellent flow in the left subclavian vein (Figure 16.4). The patient was placed on aspirin and clopidogrel instead of Coumadin warfarin, and will be followed by ultrasonographic evaluation.

References

1. Horattas MC, Wright DJ, Fenton AH et al, Changing concepts of deep venous thrombosis of the upper extremity – report of a series and review of the literature. *Surgery* 1988;**104**:561–7.

2. Adams JT, DeWeese JA, Mahoney EB et al, Intermittent subclavian vein obstruction without thrombosis. *Surgery* 1968;**63**:147–65.

3. AbuRahma AF, Robinson PA, Effort subclavian vein thrombosis: evolution of management. *J Endovasc Ther* 2000;**7**:302–8.

4. Beygui RE, Olcott C 4th, Dalman RL, Subclavian vein thrombosis: outcome analysis based on etiology and modality of treatment. *Ann Vasc Surg* 1997;**11**:247–55.

67

II STENTS, GRAFTS AND COVERED STENTS

CASE 17: THE COVERED STENT GRAFT: TREATMENT OF AN ARTERIOVENOUS FISTULA

Richard R Heuser

Background

A 64-year old woman presented for endovascular repair of an arteriovenous (AV) fistula of the subclavian artery and vein. Her left ventricular function was normal and her coronary arteries were within normal limits. She received an implantable defibrillator for a sudden death episode. The following year the leads were revised using the excimer laser as a result of multiple twists in the electrodes. After that procedure, she complained of fatigue and dyspnea. A continuous murmur was heard over the left subclavian region. Arteriography of the left subclavian artery revealed an AV fistula (Figure 17.1). After obtaining approval for compassionate use from our Institutional Review Board and the Food and Drugs Agency (FDA), the patient underwent a procedure to exclude the AV fistula with a covered stent.

Procedure

Using a brachial approach, a 45-cm 9 Fr sheath (Brite Tip, Cordis, Miami, FL, USA) was advanced under fluoroscopy. Despite multiple angiographic studies at various angles, it was difficult to locate the origin of the AV fistula. Sequential angiograms were performed by positioning the sheath until the fistula was no longer visible. A covered stent (Jomed, Helsingbord, Sweden) was then

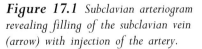

Figure 17.1 *Subclavian arteriogram revealing filling of the subclavian vein (arrow) with injection of the artery.*

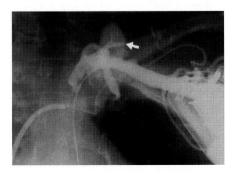

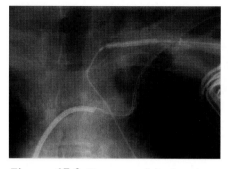

Figure 17.2 Placement of the Jomed covered stent in the subclavian.

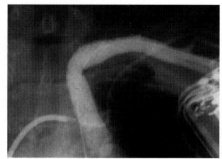

Figure 17.3 Arteriogram after deployment of the stent graft revealed exclusion of the fistula. Note that the internal mammary and vertebral arteries were excluded.

introduced to the left subclavian. As the fistula arose at the take-off point of both the vertebral and the internal mammary arteries, both were planned to be sacrificed in this patient. An earlier four-vessel study revealed that both carotids and right vertebral artery were within normal limits. After deployment of the Jomed 28-mm covered stent mounted over a 10 mm × 4 mm Opta LP balloon (Cordis, Miami, FL), we dilated the stent again with a 14 mm × 2 cm Excel balloon (SciMed/Boston Scientific, Maple Grove, MN) using 8 atm of pressure (Figure 17.2). A final angiogram showed resolution of the AV fistula (Figure 17.3). Both the vertebral and the internal mammary arteries were excluded because of the proximity of the fistula to both vessels.

Commentary

Arteriovenous fistulas are a rare but treatable cause of circulatory dysfunction and congestive heart failure. Although AV fistulas are occasionally congenital or idiopathic, they are more often associated with trauma; AV fistulas are an infrequent complication of pacemaker insertion. Clinical signs of an AV fistula may include fatigue, dyspnea and congestive heart failure, and the presence of a continuous murmur in the affected vessel. Ultimately, the lesion must be visualized angiographically to confirm the diagnosis and establish a basis for appropriate treatment. It may be difficult to locate the origin of the fistula, and sequential angiograms may be necessary.

Therapeutic approaches to correct the fistula may include open surgical intervention, balloon or coil occlusion, or use of a covered stent or endovascular graft. In our patient, a Jomed covered stent was used to correct a subclavian AV fistula with a good result. Use of a covered stent such as the Jomed allows the interventionist to perform a true internal bypass procedure using percutaneous access. The minimally invasive procedure may reduce morbidity and mortality, compared with open surgical intervention, and recovery time is generally reduced. Its use in this case allowed successful minimally invasive repair of an AV fistula, and normalized blood flow to alleviate the debilitating symptoms associated with congestive failure.

References

1. Heuser RR, Reynolds GT, Papazoglou C, Diethrich EB, Endoluminal grafting for percutaneous aneurysm exclusion in an aortocoronary saphenous vein graft: the first clinical experience. *J Endovasc Surg* 1995;**2**:81–8.

2. Anguera I, Real I, Morales M, Vazquez F, Montana X, Pare C, Left internal mammary artery to innominate vein fistula complicating pacemaker insertion. Treatment with endovascular transarterial coil embolization. *J Cardiovasc Surg (Torino)* 1999;**40**:523–5.

3. Herbreteau D, Aymard A, Khayata MH et al, Endovascular treatment of arteriovenous fistulas arising from branches of the subclavian artery. *J Vasc Interv Radiol* 1993;**4**:237–40.

4. Parodi JC, Schonholz C, Ferreira LM, Bergan J, Endovascular stent graft treatment of traumatic arterial lesions. *Ann Vasc Surg* 1999;**13**:121–9.

73

CASE 18: ENDOVASCULAR INTERVENTION FOR ACUTE AORTO-BRONCHIAL HEMORRHAGE

Larry H Hollier, Michael L Marin,
Nicholas J Morrissey, Louis DePaolo

Background

A 70-year-old man presented with hemoptysis and respiratory distress requiring intubation. Bronchoscopy documented compression and obstruction of the left main bronchus; esophagoscopy showed obstruction and esophagitis at the level of the mid-esophagus. He had sustained a type-B aortic dissection in 1997, for which he underwent open repair with a short interposition graft just beyond the left subclavian artery. He remained asymptomatic for several years until he presented with hemoptysis, and respiratory failure, and was noted to have an enlarging anastomotic pseudoaneurysm. On angiography, the type-B dissection was still evident in the descending thoracic aorta and extended to the origin of the celiac axis (Figure 18.1). A large pseudoaneurysm was evident in the upper descending thoracic aorta.

Review of computed tomography (CT) scans showed complete obstruction of the left main bronchus and opacification of the entire left lung (Figure 18.2). His clinical status was unstable and he continued to deteriorate. En route to the operating room he sustained a cardiac arrest. He was resuscitated and placed as

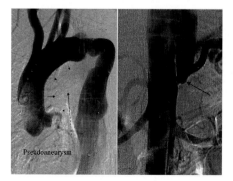

Figure 18.1 Angiogram demonstrating the previous thoracic aortic graft with persistent type-B aortic dissection that extends to the celiac axis. A large pseudoaneurysm is present medially.

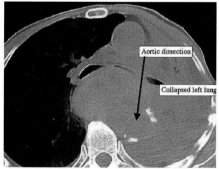

Figure 18.2 Computed tomography of the chest demonstrating compression of the left main bronchus and complete opacification of the left lung.

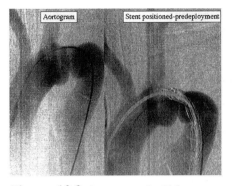

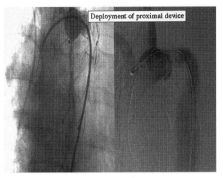

Figure 18.3 *Positioning the Talent endovascular stent graft in the aortic arch.*

Figure 18.4 *Deployment of the stent graft in the thoracic aorta, immediately distal to left carotid artery*

an emergency on the operating table with a stable, although low, blood pressure and persistent hypoxia.

Procedure

Both groins were prepped and draped. Percutaneous left femoral access was used to insert a pigtail catheter which was advanced to the ascending aortic arch. A cut-down was peformed on the right common femoral artery and a 30 mm × 20 cm Talent stent graft (Medtronic, Minneapolis, MN, USA was inserted over an 0.35-inch stiff Amplatz guidewire and positioned just distal to the left carotid artery (Figure 18.3). The graft was deployed covering the site of the proximal previous anastomosis (Figure 18.4). As the site of extravasation could not be precisely identified, two additional devices were placed to provide complete coverage of the length of dissected aorta down to and covering the origin of the celiac artery. This resulted in complete coverage of the aortobronchial fistula. Completion angiography showed no evidence of endoleak or other extravasation.

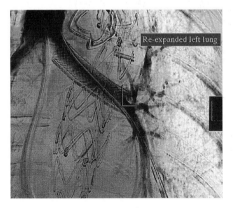

Figure 18.5 *Bronchography after placement of the bronchial stent, showing resolution of the bronchial stenosis and re-expansion of the left lung.*

75

To help resolve the patient's respiratory difficulty, a 10 mm × 4 cm Wallstent was deployed in the left main bronchus and dilated with a 10 mm balloon (Figure 18.5). This improved arterial oxygenation and allowed for re-expansion of the left lung.

Commentary

The bleeding completely resolved and the patient stabilized. However, over the next few days he was unable to be weaned from the ventilator and on postoperative day 10 a tracheostomy and feeding gastrostomy were placed. The patient remained ventilator dependent and intermittently septicemic. Ultimately the patient became profoundly hypotensive, acidotic, hypoxic and died.

Postmortem examination showed the descending thoracic aorta to be completely lined with the stent graft, with coverage of the previous aortobronchial fistula. Cultures and microscopic analysis documented nests of aspergillosis in the heart, lung, kidneys, brain and pseudoaneurysm, which had eroded into the esophagus and right bronchus.

This case illustrates that endovascular techniques are helpful in the management of acute aortobronchial fistula. However, they do not resolve any infection associated with the excluded aneurysm sac. Secondary procedures may sometimes be needed to achieve full resolution of the problems.

Case 19: Stent Graft Treatment of a Type B Aortic Dissection

Hugo Francisco Londero, Jose Norberto Allende, Francisco Eduardo Paoletti

Background

An 82-year-old woman was referred to the cardiovascular unit with a 3-day history of lumbar pain and acute leg ischemia. Blood pressure in the upper extremities was 180/90 mmHg. The left lower extremity was pale and cool and the femoral and distal pulses were absent. Right leg pulses were diminished.

Thoracic aortography through a right brachial approach demonstrated a Stanford type-B aortic dissection with the inlet in the middle third of the descending thoracic aorta (Figure 19.1). The true lumen of the infrarenal aorta was compressed and the left renal artery was poorly visualized. Spiral computed tomography (CT) confirmed the diagnosis of type-B aortic dissection. The entry site was well visualized at the midportion of the descending aorta (Figures 19.2a and 19.3a). The maximum diameter of the true lumen was 33 mm. The false lumen progressed in a retrograde fashion near the ostium of the left subclavian artery and was partially thrombosed (Figure 19.4a). The true lumen of the abdominal aorta was compressed by the false lumen (Figure 19.4a). The left

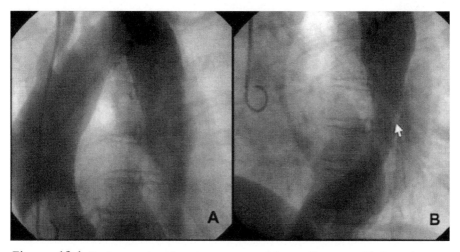

Figure 19.1 *Pre-intervention thoracic aortogram: (a) ascending aorta (b) descending aorta. Contrast filling of the false lumen began below the left subclavian artery. The arrow marks the entry site of the dissection.*

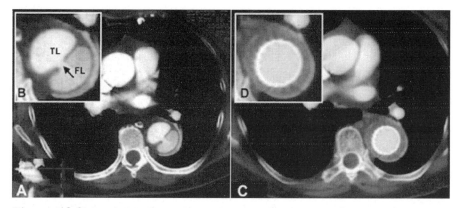

Figure 19.2 *Spiral CT scan. (a,b) Pre-intervention: the intimal flap clearly separates the true lumen (TL) and the false lumen (FL). The arrow marks the entry site of the dissection. (c,d) Post-intervention: the stent graft is uniformly expanded and completely seals the entry tear.*

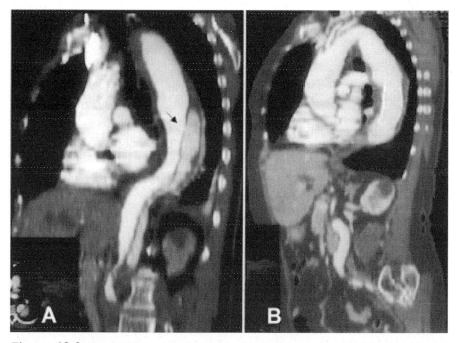

Figure 19.3 *Spiral CT scans reconstruction. (a) Pre-intervention: the false channel began below the left subclavian artery. The arrow marks the entry site of the dissection. (b) Post-intervention: the stent graft seals the entry tear.*

renal artery originated at the false lumen and the left kidney had signs of diminished perfusion (Figure 19.5b). The left iliac artery was partially occluded by compression (Figure 19.4a).

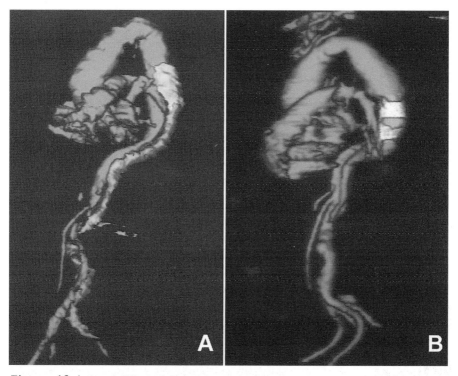

Figure 19.4 Spiral CT scan reconstruction: (a) Pre-intervention: gray — the true lumen; light gray — the false lumen. The abdominal true lumen and the left iliac are compressed and distorted. The left renal artery received the flow from the false lumen. (b) Post-intervention: white — the stent graft. The abdominal aorta and left iliac artery recovered their caliber. The left renal originates from the true lumen.

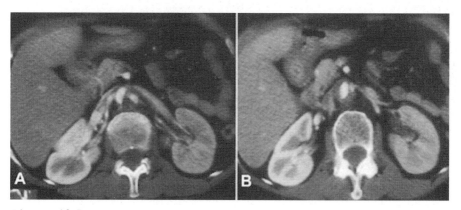

Figure 19.5 Spiral CT scans. (a) The right renal artery originates from the true lumen. (b) The left renal artery originates from the false channel.

79

The patient continued to be hospitalized and was maintained on medical treatment. Her blood pressure was controlled with propranolol and sodium nitropruside. However, she continued to have spontaneous lumbar pain and left leg claudication during ambulation, and her renal function deteriorated progressively (maximum creatinine level of 1.86 mg/dl).

Endoluminal treatment was considered and the patient's informed consent obtained. On day 22 stent graft placement was attempted.

Procedure

Under general anesthesia a right femoral artery dissection was done and a 6 Fr introducer sheath placed in the vessel. Through a 6 Fr pigtail catheter a descending thoracic aortic aortogram was performed to localize the intimal tear at the entry site (Figure 19.6a). A gauge was used as an external marker for stent graft positioning. An extra-stiff 0.035-inch wire was advanced to the ascending aorta and a 24 Fr introducer sheath (William Cook Europe A/S, Denmark) was positioned, crossing the level of the entry site.

Through the 24 Fr introducer sheath a balloon-expandable stent graft (SETA System: LATECBA SA, Buenos Aires, Argentina) was advanced to the desired

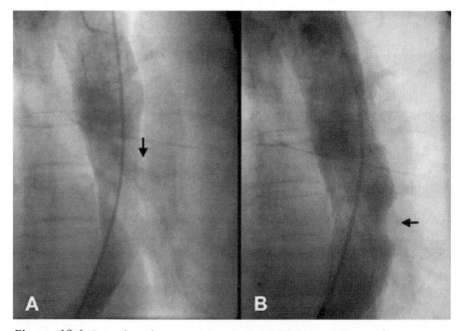

Figure 19.6 *Descending thoracic aortic angiogram. (a) Pre-intervention: the arrow marks the entry site of the dissection. The true lumen is compressed by the false channel. (b) Post-intervention: the stent graft seals the intimal tear. The graft bulges in the aortic lumen between the stents (arrow).*

level. The SETA System stent graft prosthesis is designed as follows: two giant Palmaz-type stainless steel stents at its ends act as a fixation system; they are covered with a compliant tubular knitted fabric graft. The unexpanded stents are 35 mm long and 6 mm in diameter. The graft is 80 mm in length and 26 mm in diameter when unexpanded and can be expanded up to 35 mm. The prosthesis is mounted on a 35-mm diameter/60-mm-long balloon and covered with a 21 Fr polyethylene delivery system.

Once the prosthesis reached the desired position in relation to the external gauge marker (Figure 19.7a) the cover sheath was retrieved. Thereafter the 24 Fr introducer sheath was retrieved near the proximal end of the stent graft (the introducer sheath facilitates the stent graft delivery system introduction and avoids prosthesis displacement; otherwise it anchors the system and prevents its movement during balloon inflation). Before proceeding with balloon inflation, the anesthetist maintained the mean blood pressure at less than 70 mmHg. The balloon was manually inflated with a diluted solution of ionic contrast medium and saline (Figure 19.7b). The balloon was 60 mm long, 20 mm shorter than the stent graft, to allow the expansion of the central portion of the prosthesis first, and thus avoiding Dacron folding by the sand-clock effect. The balloon must be inflated twice, distally and proximally, to expand the prosthesis completely (Figure 19.7c). A 35-mm-diameter balloon was selected to match the diameter of the aortic true lumen measured on computed tomography. A final angiogram was obtained demonstrating the complete sealing of the entry site by the stent graft (Figure 19.6b).

The patient continued in hospital 4 days after the procedure. She recovered the left leg pulses and the creatinine level dropped to 0.86 mg/dl. The post-intervention spiral CT scan demonstrated the entry to be completely sealed by

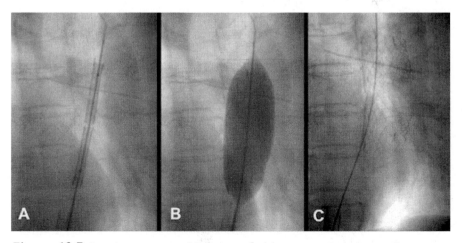

Figure 19.7 Intervention image. (a) Stent graft delivery system in place, to be expanded. Note the transversal black line corresponding to the gauge taken as an external marker. (b) Delivery balloon expanded. (c) Expanded giant Palmaz-type stents.

the prosthesis (Figures 19.2b and 19.3b). The compression of the true lumen of the abdominal aorta disappeared, despite a persistent hematoma, and normal flow was restored to the left iliac artery (Figures 19.8b and Figure 19.4b). The left renal artery originated now from the true lumen and the kidney perfusion looked normal (Figure 19.8b).

Commentary

Endovascular treatment of type-B aortic dissections and their ischemic complications is possible using different techniques. Percutaneous balloon fenestration of the intimal flap decompresses a hypertensive false lumen, collapsing the true lumen. True lumen stenting can recover aortic caliber. Selective stenting can open obstructed visceral arteries.

Endovascular sealing of the intimal tear by a stent graft decreases the tension of the false lumen, so that the blood flow through it will cease. Consequently, the false lumen is obliterated with thrombus, preventing true lumen compression and aneurysm expansion.

Left iliac flow recovery, in this particular case, may be related to true lumen decompression. More difficult to explain are the changes in the left renal circulation.

The pre-treatment spiral CT scan clearly showed that the left renal artery originated in the false lumen and the kidney was hypoperfused. After treatment, the artery originated in the true lumen and the kidney recovered its normal perfusion.

The blood pressure and the flow in the false lumen dropped by sealing the entry site of the dissection with the stent graft. These phenomena allow true lumen re-expansion. As a consequence the intimal flap was displaced, relocating the origin of the renal artery at the true lumen and re-establishing artery flow

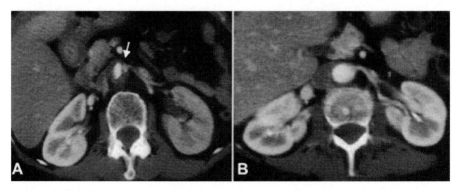

Figure 19.8 Spiral CT scans. (a) Pre-intervention: the left renal artery originates from the false lumen (arrow). The left kidney shows signs of hypoperfusion. (b) Post-intervention: the left renal artery originates from the true lumen. Left renal perfusion looks normal.

and visceral perfusion. We conclude that type-B aortic dissection, complicated with renal and lower limb ischemia, can be treated by sealing the dissection entry site with a stent graft, with improved visceral and lower extremity perfusion.

References

1. Walker PJ, Dake MD, Mitchell RS et al, The use of endovascular techniques for the treatment of complications of aortic dissection. *J Vasc Surg* 1993;**18**:1042–51.

2. Slonim SM, Nyman U, Semba CP et al, Aortic dissection: Percutaneous management of ischemic complications with endovascular stents and balloon fenestration. *J Vasc Surg* 1996;**23**:241–51.

3. Rousseau H, Otal P, Soula P et al, Diagnosis and endovascular treatment of thoracic aortic diseases. *J Radiol* 1999;**80**:1064–79.

4. Williams DM, Lee DY, Hamilton BH et al, The dissected aorta: percutaneous treatment of ischemic complications – principles and results. *J Vasc Interv Radiol* 1997;**8**:605-25.

5. Slonim SM, Myman UR, Semba CP et al, True lumen obliteration in complicated aortic dissection: endovascular treatment. *Radiology* 1996;**201**:161–6.

6. Chang WT, Kao HL, Liau CS, Lee YT, Aortic stenting on a Type B aortic dissection with visceral and limb ischemia. *Cathet Cardiovasc Intervent* 2001;**52**:112–15.

7. Nienaber CA, Fattori R, Lung G, et al, Nonsurgical reconstruction of thoracic aortic dissection by stent graft placement. *N Engl J Med* 1999;**340**:1539–45.

CASE 20: ENDOVASCULAR ABDOMINAL AORTIC ANEURYSM REPAIR WITH SUPRARENAL AORTIC FIXATION

John W York, Samuel R Money

Background

A 79-year-old man with a history of chronic obstructive pulmonary disease (COPD) and right lung lobectomy, underwent magnetic resonance imaging (MRI) of the spine after a fall and was found to have an abdominal aortic aneurysm (AAA). He subsequently underwent computed tomography (CT) of the abdomen and pelvis which confirmed an infrarenal AAA measuring 7.0 cm × 7.0 cm.

Procedure

A CT scan of the abdomen and pelvis at 3-mm intervals demonstrates a 7.0 cm × 7.0 cm infrarenal AAA (Figure 20.1). The origin of the AAA is approximately 22 mm below the level of the lowest renal artery. The maximum diameter of

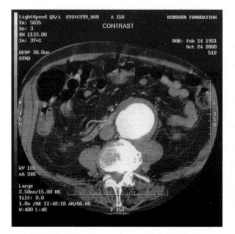

Figure 20.1 Computed tomography of the abdomen and pelvis at 3-mm intervals demonstrates a 7.0 cm × 7.0 cm infrarenal AAA.

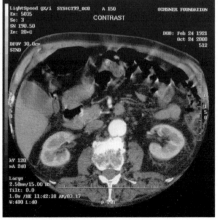

Figure 20.2 The maximum diameter of the aortic neck below the renal arteries was measured at 26 mm.

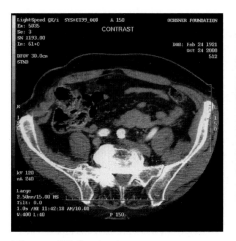

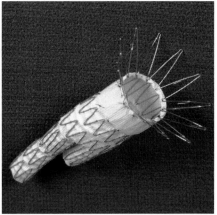

Figure 20.3 *The iliac arteries were found to be normal diameter, measuring 13 mm and 15 mm respectively*

Figure 20.4 *Zenith endovascular graft (main body) with suprarenal fixation system.*

the aortic neck below the renal arteries was measured at 26 mm (Figure 20.2). The iliac arteries were found to be normal diameter, measuring 13 mm and 15 mm respectively (Figure 20.3). The anatomy of this aneurysm seen on CT scan meets the criteria for endovascular AAA repair. Specifically, there is adequate length of non-aneurysmal aorta below the renal arteries to anchor the graft proximally, the diameter of the aortic neck is not too large to achieve an adequate seal, and the iliac arteries are of sufficient size to accept the delivery sheaths, without large aneurysmal dilatation

There was no indication for a preoperative angiogram in this case. Computed tomography is the most appropriate diagnostic imaging modality for aortic aneurysms. Although aortograms provide meaningful information about branch vessel anatomy, the technique does not accurately reflect the true anatomy of aortic aneurysms. Angiograms depict the contrast-enhanced lumen of the aorta rather than the actual size and extent of the total aneurysm.

The primary interest regarding this case is the use of an experimental endovascular AAA repair system with unique design, incorporating a suprarenal proximal aortic attachment mechanism that is self-expanding (Figures 20.4–20.6). The endovascular devices that are commercially available for AAA have specific individual design flaws, which have led to acute graft limb occlusion or endograft migration. The device used in this case is a modular system consisting of three individual elements (main body, contralateral iliac limb and ipsilateral iliac limb). It also uses a system of uncovered struts with barbs on the proximal end of the main body for suprarenal fixation (Figure 20.7). This third-generation device with enhanced modular design and suprarenal fixation may solve the problems of limb occlusion and graft migration that have been seen with the earlier device designs (Figures 20.8–20.11).

85

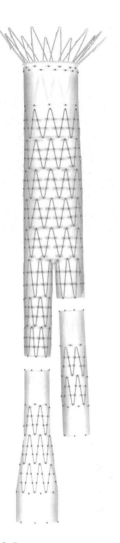

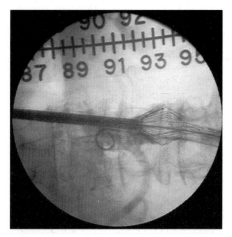

Figure 20.6 *Initial deployment of the Zenith device (main body) below the lowest renal artery.*

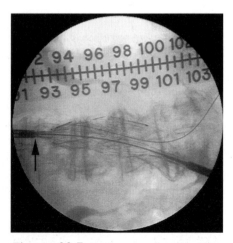

Figure 20.5 *Individual elements of the Zenith endovascular AAA repair system.*

Figure 20.7 *Deployment of suprarenal struts for proximal aortic fixation.*

Commentary

Parodi of Buenos Aires reported the first successful endovascular repair of an AAA in 1991.[1] As the experience with endovascular AAA repair has increased, several problems with this technique have been identified, which have ultimately resulted in modifications and improvements in endovascular AAA therapy.

Several problems unique to endovascular AAA repair are associated with the proximal attachment of the endograft to the native, infrarenal aorta. A primary problem is the result of the morphologic change in the aortic neck proximal to

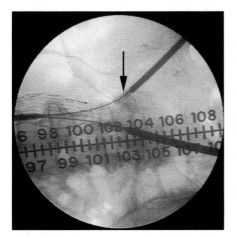

Figure 20.8 *Contralateral (left) graft limb deployment.*

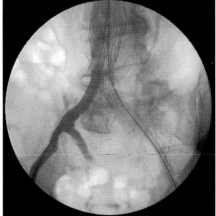

Figure 20.9 *Angiogram of right iliac artery, localizing the origin of the hypogastric artery before ipsilateral (right) graft limb deployment.*

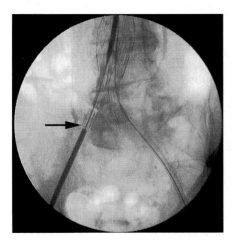

Figure 20.10 *Ipsilateral (right) graft limb deployment.*

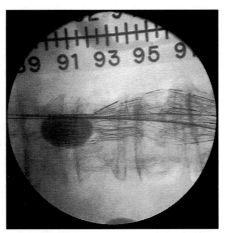

Figure 20.11 *Balloon angioplasty of the proximal aortic fixation system.*

the endovascular device, which occurs over time. After endovascular AAA repair, the segment of native infrarenal aorta has been observed to undergo progressive enlargement. This increase in diameter has been implicated in device migration and delayed appearance of blood flow within the aneurysm sac (endoleak), which may lead to aneurysm expansion and rupture (Figure 20.12).

One method of dealing with the problem of proximal aortic neck enlargement has been to over-size the proximal endograft by approximately 20%. Although this method has been reasonably effective, it is limited by the maximum diameter of available endografts in patients with a large (> 28 mm) native aorta.

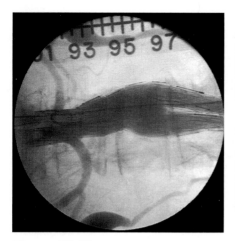 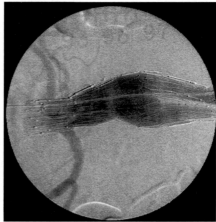

Figure 20.12 *Completion angiogram demonstrating aneurysm exclusion without evidence of endoleak.*

Figure 20.13 *Digital subtraction image showing the Gianturo Z-stent with suprarenal struts.*

Other mechanisms for proximal aortic attachment include hooks positioned on the proximal portion of the endograft and a self-expanding alloy frame that would increase in diameter as the aortic neck enlarges.

Recently, another solution to this problem has been the development of a device with suprarenal aortic fixation, as seen in the previously presented case. The Zenith (Cook Inc., Bloomington, IN, USA) endovascular stent graft uses suprarenal, uncovered struts outfitted with barbs to fix the endograft to the aortic wall. The uncovered segment of the stent graft is 22 mm in length. The infrarenal portion of the device is a woven Dacron graft supported by a self-expanding Gianturo Z-stent (Figure 20.13). As a result of the fact that the suprarenal aorta is generally less diseased than the infrarenal aorta and is not prone to enlargement, suprarenal fixation may represent an effective solution to endograft complications resulting from aortic neck enlargement. The suprarenal struts have not been shown to have a negative impact on renal artery perfusion.

Other advantages of this endograft include a self-expanding frame and modular iliac limbs. As mentioned previously, the self-expanding frame enhances the ability of the device to maintain its seal, despite enlargement of the native aorta. The advantage of the modular iliac limbs is that they allow for greater customization of the iliac portion of the endograft, based on the specific anatomic criteria of each patient.

References

1. Parodi JC, Palmaz JC, Barone HD, Transfemoral intraluminal graft implantation of abdominal aortic aneurysms. *Ann Vasc Surg* 1991;**5**:491–9.

2. Thompson MM, Boyle JR, Hartshorn T et al, Comparison of computed tomography and duplex imaging in assessing aortic morphology following endovascular repair. *Br J Surg* 1998;**85**:346–50.

3. Illig KA, Green RM, Ouriel K et al, Fate of proximal aortic cuff: Implications for endovascular aneurysm repair. *J Vasc Surg* 1997;**26**:492–501.

Case 21: Aortic stenting to seal abdominal endograft leakage

Francesco Liistro, Germano Melissano,
Antonio Colombo

Background

A 61-year-old patient with severe systemic hypertension and severe coronary artery disease treated with multiple stenting presented with an abdominal aortic aneurysm. The baseline aortogram (Figure 21.1) showed an aneurysm of the abdominal aorta which extends to the iliac arteries. The important features of this angiogram are (1) the size of the aorta at the infrarenal neck is large (24 mm) and (2) the neck below the renal arteries is very short (9 mm).

Procedure

As a result of the presence of coronary artery disease and the patient's preference, an endovascular approach was selected. Owing to the technical difficulties mentioned above, the procedure was performed using a custom-made prosthesis. A custom-made Talent endograft (32 mm × 16 mm × 14 mm + 16 mm × 8 mm) was successfully implanted with bilateral femoral cut-downs. The prosthesis was constructed with uncovered self-expanding Nitinol struts extending above the renal arteries for better anchorage of the graft to the short proximal neck.[1] At the time of implantation a small proximal endoleak was observed just below the level of the renal arteries. The leak appeared to be minor and no action was taken.

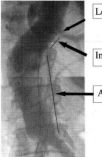

Left renal artery ostium

Infrarenal neck

Aneurismatic segment

Figure 21.1 *Angiography of the abdominal aorta showing the infra-renal aneurysm. Note the short infra-renal neck and the long aneurysmatic segment which extends to the iliac arteries (arrows).*

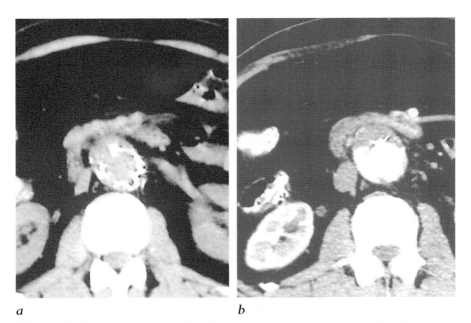

a   b

Figure 21.2 *Computed tomography of the abdominal aorta three days after the implantation of a custom-made prosthesis showing:*
(a) significant malapposition of the proximal edge of the prosthesis to the aortic wall.
(b) incomplete exclusion of the aneurysm by contrast medium injection.

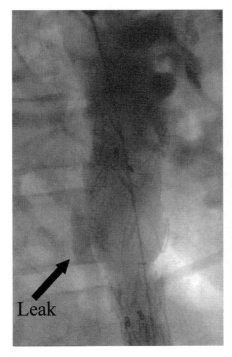

Figure 21.3 *Repeated angiography of the treated aneurysmatic segment which shows:*
(a) significant leak at the proximal edge of the prosthesis with contrast medium seen behind the prosthesis struts.
(b) ultrasound evaluation of the proximal edge of the prosthesis showing the irregular contour and the incomplete apposition to the aortic wall.

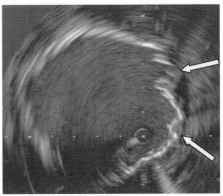

a   b

Follow-up computed tomography 3 days after the procedure is shown in Figure 21.2, which demonstrates significant malapposition of the proximal edge of the prosthesis to the aortic wall (Figure 21.2a) with incomplete exclusion of the aneurysm (Figure 21.2b). For this reason we decided to perform a new aortogram and intravascular ultrasound (IVUS) in order to resolve the proximal endoleak.[2] Figure 21.3a shows the angiographic image of the prominent proximal leak, with contrast seen behind the proximal end of the prosthesis and Figure 21.3b shows the IVUS image obtained with a 12.5-MHz Medi-Tech catheter (Boston Scientific Corp., Watertown, MA, USA) at the level of the proximal neck, showing the irregular contour and the incomplete apposition of the prosthesis to the aortic wall.

An attempt was made to expand further the prosthesis with a 28 mm × 50 mm Cristal balloon (Balt Extrusion, Montmorency, France) at 4 atm (Figure 21.4a). An angiography (Figure 21.4b) and ultrasound evaluation (Figure 21.4c) following balloon inflation did not show resolution of the endoleak and the prosthesis still appeared asymmetrically expanded. For this reason it was decided to seal the proximal leak with a P5014 Palmaz stent (Cordis, Miami, FL), to be positioned across the proximal end of the prosthesis for better anchorage of the whole device to the aortic wall and complete exclusion of the aneurysm.

A Palmaz stent was hand mounted on a 28 mm × 50 mm balloon and inserted into the right femoral artery using a 14 Fr sheath. The stent was expanded at 6 atm. to straddle the graft across the origin of the renal arteries. Figure 21.5 shows the stent implantation (Figure 21.5a), final angiogram (Figure 21.5b) and

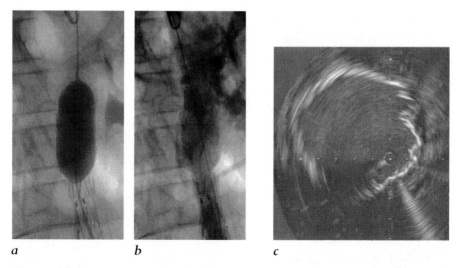

a   *b*   *c*

Figure 21.4 *(a) Balloon dilatation of the proximial edge of the prosthesis with a 28 × 50 mm balloon. (b) Persistent leak image after balloon dilatation. (c) Persistent irregular contour of the proximal edge of the prosthesis by ultrasound evaluation after balloon dilatation.*

92

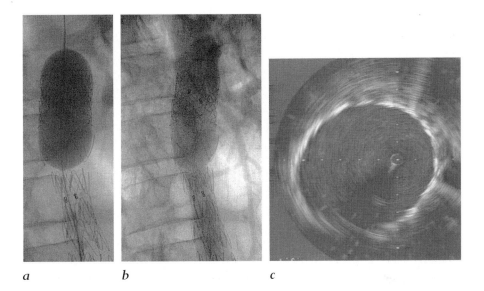

a   b   c

Figure 21.5 *Palmaz stent implantation at the proximal edge of the prosthesis:*
(a) Palmaz stent pre-mounted on a 28 × 50 mm balloon implanted at a pressure of 6 atmospheres
(b) angiographic resolution of the leak after stent implantation
(c) regular prosthesis contour with complete apposition of the struts to the aortic wall and wide circular aortic lumen by post-stenting ultrasound evaluation.

IVUS evaluation (Figure 21.5c) which demonstrate complete sealing of the proximal endoleak with symmetric and full expansion of the prosthesis. Figure 21.6 shows the stent struts expanded over the proximal end of the Talent endograft. The intraprosthesis cross-sectional area was 506 mm^2 after balloon dilatation and 728 mm^2 after stent deployment. The patient recovered uneventfully and was discharged 5 days later.

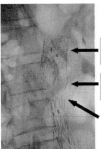

Balloon expandable
Palmaz stent

Uncovered initial struts
of the prosthesis

Covered proximal
end of the prosthesis

Figure 21.6 *Stent struts expanded over the proximal edge of the prosthesis.*

93

Commentary

This case illustrates the possibility of correcting an endoleak using a percutaneous approach.[3] A tortuous and irregular aorta at the level of a short proximal neck may be an insufficient landing point even for a custom-made self-expanding, partially covered prosthesis designed to straddle the renal arteries. The force created by the self-expanding stent struts may be insufficient to anchor the prosthesis fully on the short and asymmetric neck.[4] The availability of a balloon-expandable stent such as the Palmaz for better anchorage of the device is a reasonable alternative. This Palmaz stent is labelled by the manufacturer as having an expansion range up to 25 mm at 2 atm. In this specific case, the size of the proximal end of the aneurysmatic segment evaluated by IVUS was 28.4 mm and the final size of the dilated stent was 31.9 mm. This fact supports the concept of using IVUS for better identification of the optimal size of the device to use and the fact that this type of stent may be dilated above its nominal size.

References

1. Greenberg R, Fairman R, Srivastava S, Criado F, Green R, Endovascular grafting in patients with short proximal necks: an analysis of short-term results. *Cardiovasc Surg* 2000;**8**:350–4.

2. Wain RA, Marin ML, Ohki T et al, Endoleaks after endovascular graft treatment of aortic aneurysms: classification, risk factors, and outcome. *J Vasc Surg* 1998;**27**:69–78; discussion 78–80.

3. Jacobowitz GR, Rosen RJ, Riles TS, The significance and management of the leaking endograft. *Semin Vasc Surg* 1999;**12**:199–206.

4. Laheij RJ, Buth J, Harris PL, Moll FL, Stelter WJ, Verhoeven EL, Need for secondary interventions after endovascular repair of abdominal aortic aneurysms. intermediate-term follow-up results of a European collaborative registry. *Br J Surg* 2000;**87**:1666–73.

CASE 22: PERCUTANEOUS ENDOVASCULAR TREATMENT OF RUPTURED ABDOMINAL AORTIC ANEURYSM

Edward B Diethrich, Julio A Rodriguez,
Venkatesh Ramaiah, Charles Thompson

Background

An 85-year-old woman in frail health was admitted to the hospital for lethargy and abdominal pain. She was hypotensive and had a pulsatile abdominal mass. Computed tomography (CT) of the abdomen revealed an 8-cm ruptured infrarenal abdominal aortic aneurysm. The patient adamantly refused open resection, but consented to endovascular treatment.

Procedure

The admission CT scan (Figure 22.1) showed an 8-cm ruptured aortic aneurysm with retroperitoneal hemorrhage. The patient was expeditiously taken to an operating room fully equipped with angiographic and fluoroscopic equipment. Angiography (Figure 22.2) revealed a 2-cm proximal neck with extravasation of contrast. The iliac arteries were of normal caliber and free of atherosclerotic disease.

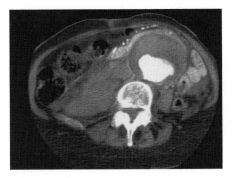

Figure 22.1 Computed tomography of a ruptured infrarenal aortic aneurysm with prominent retroperitoneal hematoma.

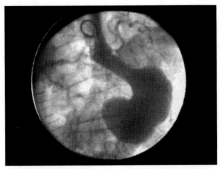

Figure 22.2 Angiography showing an 8-cm aneurysm, with a 2-cm proximal neck.

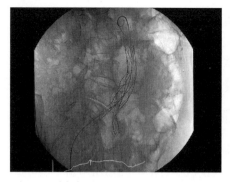

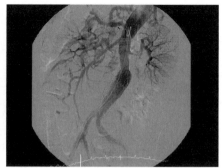

Figure 22.3 *Fully deployed Endologix bifurcated graft.*

Figure 22.4 *Post-deployment angiography showing positioning below the renal arteries and exclusion of the aneurysm.*

Under minimal sedation, a bifurcated unibody endograft (Endologix: Phoenix, AZ, USA) was deployed percutaneously via a 12 Fr sheath in the right common femoral artery and a 9 Fr sheath in the left common femoral artery. The proximal end of the device was positioned below the renal arteries, and the limbs were deployed below the bifurcation in the common iliac arteries (Figure 22.3). A completion angiogram visualized both renal arteries and demonstrated good exclusion of the aneurysm without endoleaks (Figure 22.4). The right delivery sheath was removed and the vessel was closed with a fascia suture. The contralateral sheath was removed and groin pressure applied.

Deployment of the device took 40 min, and the entire procedure lasted 90 min. Procedure-related blood loss was less than 100 ml, and the patient received 4 units of peripheral red blood cells during the procedure. Approximately 300 ml of contrast was used. Upon transfer to the recovery room, the patient was awake and in a stable condition.

Postoperatively, the patient remained hemodynamically stable. An abdominal CT scan on postoperative day 1 showed a successfully excluded aneurysm with no endoleak (Figure 22.5).

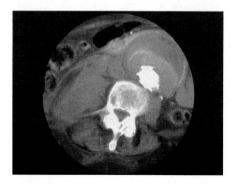

Figure 22.5 *Postprocedural CT scan of the Endologix graft without endoleak.*

The patient was ambulating and tolerating regular diet by postoperative day 2. The patient was discharged shortly thereafter and had an uneventful recovery.

Commentary

Rupture is a highly lethal complication of an abdominal aortic aneurysm. Many patients (50%) die before they reach a medical facility. If they reach the operating room, the operative mortality rate is 50%. The overall mortality rate of ruptured abdominal aortic aneurysms is therefore between 75% and 90%.[1,2] In the face of such dramatic mortality, the repair of ruptured aneurysms with endoluminal grafts appears to be profoundly controversial. However, the nature of the rupture affects mortality. Those who present with free peritoneal rupture have a mortality rate that is over 90%, whereas those who have a contained leak have a mortality rate of less than 20%.[1] Given the success of elective endovascular stent graft repair of aneurysms, similar repair of ruptured aneurysms presents an interesting option, particularly in those with contained leaks.

The mainstay of prevention of aneurysm rupture is elective repair. Aggressive programs of elective resection have resulted in an overall decrease in the incidence of abdominal aortic aneurysm rupture. Endovascular techniques are now commonly employed to repair aneurysms electively and have expanded our ability to treat high risk surgical patients. Endovascular repair of ruptured aneurysms has met a more tempered enthusiasm, mainly because of perceived difficulties with preoperative measurement, device procurement and longer times to obtain hemodynamic control. The technique of ruptured aneurysm endovascular repair is still in its infancy and has been embraced cautiously.[3–8] The standard by which we are judged remains open resection and, as any surgeon will attest, it is a complex and challenging procedure in the face of rupture.

Certain advantages to the endovascular approach in the repair of a ruptured abdominal aortic aneurysm cannot be overlooked. The ability to access a site distal to the rupture and avoid the retroperitoneal dissection is the most obvious. Elimination of the technical difficulties of open resection brought about by hemorrhage, and distortion of retroperitoneal structures by hematoma, is sufficient cause to consider endovascular stent grafting.[3,6] Maintenance of hemodynamic stability by the avoidance of prolonged intraoperative hypotension is a major determinant of postoperative outcome and directly impacts on survival.[9] We certainly feel that, in many cases, initial aortic control can be quickly obtained with an aortic balloon faster and more safely than open dissection and cross-clamp. Endovascular repair also has less blood loss compared with open procedures, and prefabricated bifurcated systems allow for rapid deployment. The result is a more controlled procedure without wide variations in blood pressure and a potentially better outcome.

97

This patient with a ruptured 8-cm aneurysm who refused an open surgical procedure offered the perfect opportunity to attempt endovascular repair through an entirely percutaneous approach. Our stock supply of endografts includes a variety of models and extensions. In particular, the Endologix device allows for deployment through a 12 and 9 Fr introducer sheath without femoral artery cut-down. If the aneurysm morphology allows for endovascular repair according to the specifications of the device, we believe that prefabricated devices can be successfully used in the treatment of ruptured aneurysm, as this case successfully illustrates.

References

1. Bickerstaff LK, Hollier LH, Van Peenen HJ, Melton LJ III, Pairolero PC, Cherry KJ, Abdominal aortic aneurysms: the changing natural history. *J Vasc Surg* 1984;**1**:6–12.

2. Taylor LM Jr, Porter JM, Basic data related to clinical decision-making in abdominal aortic aneurysms. *Ann Vasc Surg* 1987;**1**:502–4.

3. Ohki T, Veith FJ, Sanchez LA et al, Endovascular graft repair of ruptured aortoiliac aneurysms. *J Am Coll Surg* 1999;**189**:102-113.

4. Greenberg RK, Srivastava SD, Ouriel K et al, An endoluminal method of hemorrhage control and repair of ruptured abdominal aortic aneurysms. *J Endovasc Ther* 2000;**7**:1–7.

5. Seelig MH, Berchtold C, Jakob P et al, Contained rupture of an infrarenal abdominal aortic aneurysm treated by endoluminal repair. *Eur J Vasc Endovasc Surg* 2000;**19**:202–4.

6. Ohki T, Veith FJ, Endovascular grafts and other image-guided catheter-based adjuncts to improve the treatment of ruptured aortoiliac aneurysms. *Ann Surg* 2000;**232**:466–79.

7. Schönholz C, Donnini F, Naselli G, Pocovi A, Parodi JC, Acute rupture of an aortic false aneurysm treated with a stent-graft. *J Endovasc Surg* 1999;**6**:293–6.

8. Umscheid T, Stelter WJ, Endovascular treatment of an aortic aneurysm ruptured into the inferior vena cava. *J Endovasc Ther* 2000;**7**:31–5.

9. Sasaki S, Yasuda K, Yamauchi H, Shiiya N, Sakuma M, Determinants of postoperative and long-term survival of patients with ruptured abdominal aortic aneurysms. *Surg Today* 1998;**28**:30–5.

CASE 23: RHEOLYTIC THROMBECTOMY FOR AORTIC ENDOGRAFT THROMBOSIS

Zvonimir Krajcer

Background

A 77-year-old man presented 1 month after abdominal aortic aneurysm (AAA) repair using an Ancure endograft with rest pain and absent lower extremity (LE) pulses.

Procedure

Angiography revealed thrombosed endograft (Figure 23.1). Successful thrombectomy of the endograft with reconstitution of the arterial flow (Figure 23.2) was achieved with Angiojet Xpeedior (Figure 23.3) catheter. The cause of thrombosis was kinking and external compression of the iliac limbs. This problem was corrected with repeat angioplasty and re-stenting of the iliac limbs.

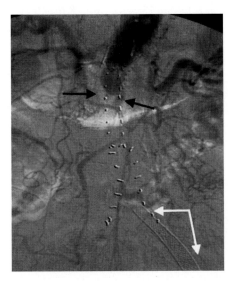

Figure 23.1 *Angiography via the left brachial artery shows complete occlusion of the endograft (black arrows) just below the renal arteries. The Wallstent can be seen in the left iliac limb (white arrows).*

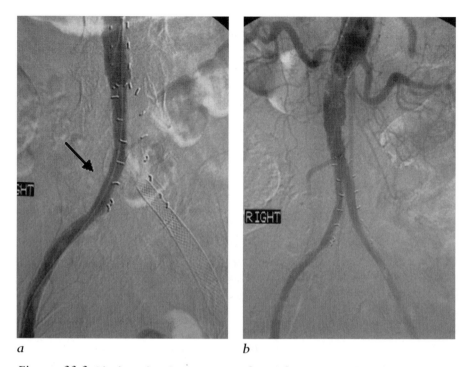

a   b

Figure 23.2 *Rheolytic thrombectomy was performed first on the right limb (a) (arrows) and then on the left limb (b), both from the anterograde brachial artery cut-down approach.*

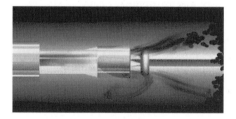

Figure 23.3 *The Angiojet Xpeedior catheter has tiny holes spaced evenly around the ring. High-speed saline jets create a low-pressure zone inside the vessel, which in turn creates a 360° Bernoulli effect. This attracts thrombus around the catheter tip for rapid removal.*

Commentary

One complication of endovascular repair of AAA is endograft thrombosis. This case illustrates the problem of thrombosis that is not infrequently encountered with current generation endografts. In contrast to supported endografts, the Ancure device is a unibody, unsupported, polyester graft with metallic attachment hooks at the proximal aortic end and at both iliac ends. Unsupported endograft material is susceptible to kinking and extrinsic compression. This commonly occurs at sites of severe angulation. The unibody design also predisposes limbs to twist, leading to decreased blood flow and resulting in endograft thrombosis. To prevent this, angioplasty and stenting in iliac limbs are frequently done. Amesur et al[2] reported that 46% of their patients in whom

Ancure was used required stenting to resolve this problem. He further reported that 17% developed thrombosis of the iliac limbs at follow-up.

Extrinsic compression and kinking had occurred in our patient at the time of the Ancure endograft deployment. This was corrected with angioplasty and stenting with a Wallstent (Boston Scientific, Watertown, MA, USA). Even though satisfactory angiographic results were achieved, this patient ultimately developed thrombosis, in spite of anticoagulation with warfarin (Coumadin) for the treatment of chronic atrial fibrillation.

The principal goal of treatment of acute LE ischemia is rapid restoration of blood flow to the ischemic region before irreversible changes occur. There are several options available for treating thrombosed endografts, including Fogarty embolectomy, thrombolysis and thrombectomy devices.

Fogarty embolectomy has been reported to be effective in treating limb thrombosis. This procedure is not, however, without risks, and involves surgery and general anesthesia. Thrombolysis is another method of treating thrombosed endografts if the occlusion is detected early and LEs are not threatened. Approximately 20% of patients have contraindications to thrombolytic therapy.

A number of mechanical devices have been developed to disrupt and remove freshly formed thrombus from the arterial circulation. Rheolytic thrombectomy is of most value when used to remove thrombi that are of recent onset. Thrombus is removed by generating a Bernoulli effect-induced vacuum at the tip of the catheter, pulling thrombus into the heparinized saline stream, which results in micro-fragmentation. Micro-fragments are discharged through the outflow lumen into the collecting bag. Wagner et al[6] reported the success rate of 90% and low incidence of amputation and mortality when using rheolytic thrombectomy for treatment of limb ischemia. Angiojet catheters were first designed for coronary vessels; they are the size of 5 Fr, requiring a 0.018-inch guidewire. The second-generation Angiojet device (Xpeedior) is 6 Fr in size and compatible with a 0.035-inch wire, offering greater effectiveness in thrombus removal and better suited for treating larger peripheral vessels.

In this case, we chose rheolytic thrombectomy because it offered rapid and effective restoration of blood flow to the LEs. This was achieved faster than could have been achieved with thrombolysis. This approach also avoided the risks involved with surgery and general anesthesia, and the need for a Fogarty embolectomy. Endograft procedures are rapidly increasing in the USA. Rheolytic thrombectomy may become a valuable tool in the treatment of endograft thrombosis.

References

1. Moore WS, Rutherford RB, for the EVT Investigators, Transfemoral endovascular repair of abdominal aortic aneurysm. Results of the North American EVT, phase I trial. *J Vasc Surg* 1996;2:543–53.

101

2. Amesur NB, Zajko AB, Orons PD, Makaroun MS, Endovascular treatment of iliac limb stenosis or occlusions in 31 patients treated with the Ancure endograft. *J Vasc Intervent Radiol* 2000;**11**:421–8.

3. Amesur NB, Zajko AB, Makaroun MS, Treatment of failed bifurcated abdominal aortic stent graft with thrombolysis and Wallstent placement. *J Vasc Intervent Radiol* 1997;**8**:795–8.

4. May J, White GH, Yu W et al, Surgical management of complications following endoluminal grafting of abdominal aortic aneurysms. *Eur J Vasc Endovasc Surg* 1995;**10**:51–9.

5. Silva TA, Ramee SR, Collins TJ et al, Rheolytic thrombectomy in the treatment of acute limb-threatening ischemia: immediate results and six-month follow-up of the multi-center angio-jet registry. Possis peripheral Angiojet study investigators. *Cathet Cardiovasc Diag* 1998;**45**:386–92.

6. Wagner HY, Muller-Hulsbeck S et al, Rapid thrombectomy with hydrodynamic catheter: Results from a prospective multi-center trial. *Radiology* 1997;**205**:675–81.

CASE 24: STENT GRAFT PLACEMENT FOR ILIAC ARTERY ANEURYSM

S Jody Stagg III, Peter Fail

Background

The patient is a 83-year-old man with a history of coronary artery disease (CAD), congestive heart failure (CHF), severe chronic obstructive pulmonary disease (COPD), carotid artery disease and chronic atrial fibrillation. Peripheral angiography performed for claudication and decreased ankle brachial indices (ABIs) demonstrated a large isolated iliac artery aneurysm of the left common iliac artery (Figure 24.1). As a result of the patient's severe COPD and other co-morbidities it was felt that surgical repair carried a prohibitively high risk. Therefore, endoluminal treatment with a covered WallGraft was proposed.

Procedure

Informed consent for this investigational procedure was obtained. The left femoral artery was entered in a retrograde fashion. The iliac aneursym was crossed with a Terumo glidewire (Boston Scientific, Watertown, MA, USA) and then exchanged for an extra-support 0.035-inch guidewire. A 12 mm × 70 mm WallGraft (Boston Scientific) was deployed without difficulty. It appeared that there was adequate apposition and adherence to the short proximal neck of the common iliac (Figure 24.2a).

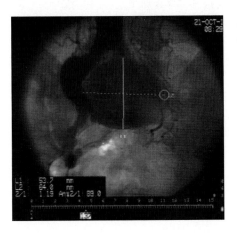

Figure 24.1 *Isolated iliac artery aneursym measuring 5.3 cm − 6.4 cm.*

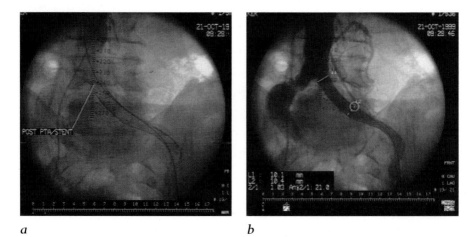

a   *b*

Figure 24.2 *(a) Post deployment of covered Wallgraft. (b) Angiogram post deployment with small endo leak.*

Post-deployment angiography demonstrated the WallGraft to be in good position with slight extravasation of contrast through the graft material (Figure 24.2b). This was expected to resolve with time. At the 3-month follow-up visit, a left lower quadrant pulsatile mass, which had resolved immediately after the procedure, was again present. Computed tomography (CT) of the abdomen confirmed the prolapse of the WallGraft into the body of the aneurysm. Repeat angiography demonstrated the proximal end of the WallGraft to be in the midportion of the aneurysm (Figure 24.3).

Re-intervention was performed after having obtained approval from the patient, IRB, and the trial sponsor. The WallGraft was crossed with a floppy wire, which was then snared from the contralateral right femoral approach and pulled into the distal aorta (Figure 24.4). An additional WallGraft was then

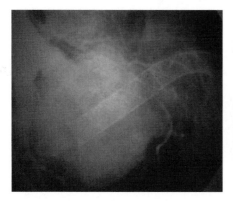

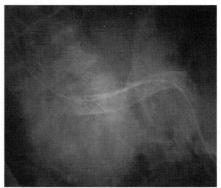

Figure 24.3 *Six-month follow-up demonstrating graft migration into aneursym.*

Figure 24.4 *Graft re-wired in a retrograde fashion*

104

deployed in the distal aorta and proximal left common iliac. A WallGraft was also placed on the right side to provide contralateral support, to prevent compromise of the right common iliac and to exclude a smaller right iliac aneurysm (Figure 24.5).

Final angiography demonstrated complete exclusion of the left iliac aneurysm with minimal contrast 'leak' through the graft material (Figure 24.6). This was not considered to be an endoleak. On the 3-month follow-up examination, the palpable left lower quadrant mass was no longer present. The 6-month CT scan of the abdomen demonstrated a very small endoleak on the right side, with complete exclusion of the left iliac aneurysm.

Commentary

Isolated iliac artery aneurysms (IAAs) are rare. In patients with abdominal aortic aneurysm (AAA), involvement of the iliac arteries has been reported to be as high as 50%. In postmortem studies, the incidence of an AAA is reported to be 3.8%. Isolated IAA incidence varies between 0.03% and 0.1%. Predicting rupture has been difficult. Compounding the problem is the consequence of rupture. IAA rupture is associated with a mortality rate of up to 80%. Dobrin[6] reported that 36% of patients with an isolated IAA will experience expansion. The average rate of expansion was 4 mm/year. In hopes of preventing the dire effect of rupture, intervention is frequently indicated. Conventional therapy has consisted of surgical reconstruction with graft interposition. Perioperative mortality rates as high as 13% are associated with surgical repair. This has been the stimulus driving the development of less invasive alternatives, including endovascular repair with a variety of covered stents.

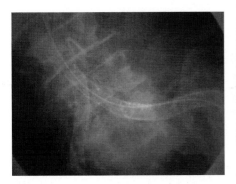

Figure 24.5 *Placement of Wallgrafts placed at the common iliac bifurcation.*

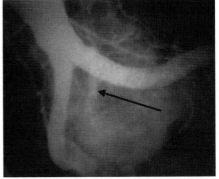

Figure 24.6 *Angiogram after iliac bifurcation reconstruction with exclusion of aneurysm. Arrow depicts small endoleak on the left which was absent on the 3-month CT scan.*

References

1. Richardson JW, Greenfield LJ, Natural history and management of iliac aneurysms. *J Cardiovas Surg* 1992;**33**:679–83.

2. Brukwall J, Hauksson H, Bengtsson H et al, Solitary aneurysms of the iliac arterial system; an estimate of their frequency and occurrence. *J Vasc Surg* 1989;**10**:381–4.

3. Lucke B, Rea MH, Studies on aneurysm. *JAMA* 1921;**77**:935–40.

4. Kunz R. Aneurysmata bei 35380 Autosien. *Schweiz Med Wochenschr* 1980;**110**:142–8.

5. Bolin T, Lund K, Slau T, Isolated aneurysms of the iliac artery: what are the chances of rupture? *Eur J Vasc Surg* 1988;**2**:213–15.

6. Dobrin PB, Mechanics of normal and diseased blood vessels. *Ann Vasc Surg* 1988;204–94.

7. Schroeder RA, Flanagan TL, Kron I et al, AA safe approach to the treatment of iliac artery aneursyms: aortobifemoral bypass grafting with exclusion of the aneurysm. *Am J Surg* 1991;**57**:624–6.

8. Scheinert D, Schroder M et al, Treatment of iliac artery aneurysm by percutaneous implantation of stent grafts. *Circulation* 2000;**102**:111–253.

III VISCERAL AND RENAL INTERVENTIONS

CASE 25: CELIAC ARTERY STENTING FOR CORONARY 'STEAL' SYNDROME

Craig Walker

Background

A 71-year-old white woman presented with exertional chest discomfort, increasing fatigue and lower extremity pain. Ten years earlier the patient received a left internal mammary artery (LIMA) bypass to the left anterior descending artery (LAD), a saphenous vein graft to the first obtuse marginal branch, and a saphenous vein graft to a large posterior lateral branch. Other pertinent features of the patient's history included bilateral carotid endarterectomy, chronic obstructive pulmonary disease, hypertension,

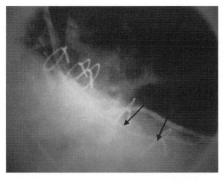

a

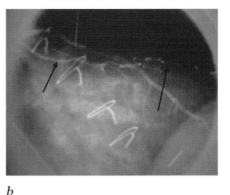

b

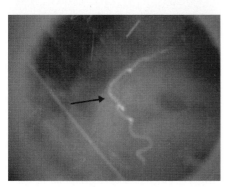

c

Figure 25.1 (a) Pericardiophrenic branch of LIMA. (b) Pericardiophrenic branch of LIMA. (c) Left gastric artery filling via pericardiophrenic branch.

neuropathy of the left lower extremity and moderate aortic stenosis (valve area of 1.4 cm^2).

A technetium [^{99m}Tc]sestamibi perfusion study suggested anterior ischemia, and coronary angiography was performed. Coronary angiography demonstrated a stenosis of 70% at the origin of the left main coronary artery and the LAD and circumflex arteries were totally occluded in their proximal portion. Vein grafts to two circumflex marginal branches were patent as was a LIMA graft to the LAD. LIMA injections demonstrated a large pericardiophrenic branch supplying collaterals to the left gastric artery (Figure 25.1). The identification of the unusually large retrograde collateral to the left gastric system via the LIMA, and the absence of other anatomic explanation for the patient's signs and symptoms, aroused suspicion of a possible coronary steal syndrome.

Procedure

The patient underwent abdominal aortography. This study demonstrated an ostial 80% celiac artery stenosis and a 90% stenosis near the origin of the superior mesenteric artery (SMA). Our approach was to correct the stenosis in the celiac axis to reduce the need for collateral flow to the left gastric artery via the LIMA. This would potentially reduce the 'coronary steal' phenomenon and improve perfusion to the celiac distribution.

The following day, the patient underwent percutaneous intervention of the celiac stenosis. The left common femoral artery was entered in a retrograde fashion. An 8 Fr renal artery guiding catheter was placed selectively into the celiac artery and a preliminary angiogram was obtained. The angiogram demonstrated a discrete, concentric stenosis of 80% at the origin of the celiac artery (Figure 25.2). This obstruction was crossed without difficulty with a 0.018-inch steerable guidewire. A 7 mm × 3 cm angioplasty balloon was placed at the origin of the celiac artery and a single dilatation at 4 atm was performed (Figure 25.3).

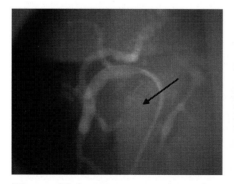

Figure 25.2 Stenosis at the origin of the celiac artery.

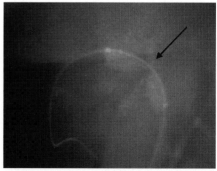

Figure 25.3 Balloon indentation by the aorto-ostial celiac artery lesion.

110

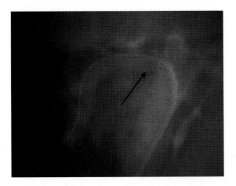

Figure 25.4 Angiography of the celiac axis origin post stent deployment.

A 16-mm Intrastent was then deployed on a 7 mm × 2 cm balloon (Figure 25.4). Good run-off was documented in the hepatic, gastric and splenic distributions of the celiac artery. The patient was discharged the next day without complications. Three-month follow-up revealed that the patient was free of angina symptoms. Non-invasive nuclear studies at 9 months were negative for ischemia.

Commentary

This case describes an unusual presentation of coronary artery steal syndrome whereby blood flow from a LIMA graft anastomosed to the LAD was partially diverted via collateral to the left gastric artery. The apparent cause of the steal syndrome, severe celiac axis stenosis, was successfully treated with percutaneous transluminal angioplasty (PTA) and stent placement.

The LIMA has proved to be an excellent conduit for myocardial revascularization in coronary bypass, and is typically anastomosed to the LAD or a diagonal branch. Ischemia of the anterior wall of the left ventricle may result if blood flow through the LIMA becomes retrograde. This can occur with subclavian stenosis. Ischemia may also result when blood is diverted, as observed when side branches of the LIMA are not ligated at the time of bypass surgery, resulting in a coronary 'steal' syndrome. The present case illustrates an example of the latter phenomenon.

Case 26: Celiac artery intervention

Christopher J White, Stephen R Ramee

Background

A 57-year-old woman with diffuse atherosclerotic coronary and peripheral vascular disease presented with progressively worsening abdominal pain, particularly after eating a meal. She had lost about 20 pounds (9 kg) over the past several months because she was avoiding meals. She was referred for diagnostic angiography, which demonstrated a 99% stenosis of the celiac artery, and occlusion of the superior mesenteric and inferior mesenteric arteries. The celiac lesion was seen only on the lateral projection.

Procedure

The right brachial artery was entered percutaneously, a 8 Fr arterial sheath placed and 5000 IU heparin were given. An 8 Fr multipurpose coronary angioplasty guiding catheter was inserted and, using the lateral view, selectively engaged the celiac artery (Figure 26.1). An exchange-length 0.014-inch Sport wire (Guidant, Temecula, CA, USA) was advanced across the lesion and into the hepatic artery. A 5 mm × 2 cm Opta-5 balloon (Cordis, Miami, FL) was advanced to the lesion and inflated at 6 atm. Post-dilatation angiography demonstrated a significant residual stenosis resulting from recoil of the ostial lesion, and the balloon was judged to be undersized. A 6 mm × 2 cm Opta-5 balloon was then used to dilate the lesion, but there continued to be evidence of significant recoil at the ostium of the vessel and a decision was made to place a stent.

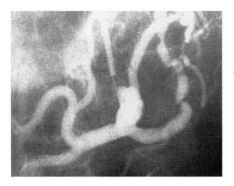

Figure 26.1 *Selective angiography of the celiac trunk, showing a 99% eccentric stenosis at the origin of the celiac artery from the aorta.*

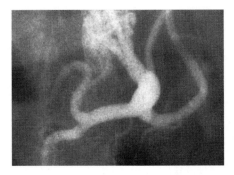

Figure 26.2 *Selective angiography after stent placement in the celiac artery with resolution of the stenosis.*

The balloon was withdrawn. A P104 (Palmaz: Cordis) stent was hand crimped on to a 6 mm × 2 cm Opta-5 balloon and advanced over the wire to the lesion and carefully positioned at the ostium. The stent was deployed at 10 atm with a 10% residual stenosis. A 7 mm × 2 cm Opta-5 balloon was used to post-dilate the stent at 12 atm with no residual stenosis (Figure 26.2).

The patient was discharged the next morning on daily aspirin 325 mg and clopidogrel (Plavix) 75 mg.

Commentary

This is a typical history of visceral ischemia — a vague aching discomfort in the abdomen — usually after eating. This patient had systemic atherosclerosis with coronary, carotid and lower extremity involvement. Patients with bowel ischemia will frequently manifest significant weight loss as a result of food avoidance. The diagnosis is usually made clinically and confirmed angiographically. Other imaging modalities such as spiral computed tomography and magnetic resonance angiography would also be helpful.

This patient illustrates the use of the brachial artery approach for engaging the mesenteric vessel and occasionally for a superiorly oriented renal artery. The greatest difficulty with this access is the use of 8 Fr sheaths and guiding catheters in the relatively small brachial artery.

CASE 27: SUPERIOR MESENTERIC ARTERY INTERVENTION (FEMORAL APPROACH)

Stephen R Ramee, Christopher J White

Background

A 71-year-old man presents with a history of abdominal cramping pain after meals associated with a weight loss of 20 pounds (9 kg) over the past 6 months. Diagnostic angiography demonstrated a critical stenosis of the proximal superior mesenteric artery (SMA) (Figure 27.1). The celiac artery was patent but the inferior mesenteric artery was occluded.

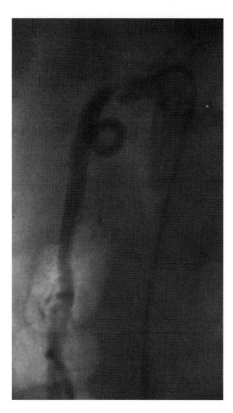

Figure 27.1 *Lateral view of a selective injection of the superior mesenteric artery with a 90% stenosis of the proximal vessel.*

Procedure

Left common femoral access was obtained, and a 6 Fr sheath was placed and 3000 IU heparin were given. A 6 Fr internal mammary artery (IMA) catheter was inserted over an exchange-length 0.035-inch Wholey (Malinckrodt, St Louis, MO, USA) guidewire. In a lateral projection, the superior mesenteric artery was engaged and a selective angiogram is shown in Figure 27.1.

The lesion was crossed with the Wholey wire and the 6 Fr sheath was exchanged for a 8 Fr sheath. The 6 Fr IMA catheter was exchanged over the wire for an 8 Fr hockey-stick guiding catheter. The lesion was pre-dilated with 5 mm × 2 cm Opta-5 (Cordis, Miami, FL) balloon. The balloon was removed and a P104 (Palmaz: Cordis) stent was hand mounted and then deployed at the lesion site. As a result of a residual stenosis of about 20%, it was elected to post-dilate the stent with a 6 mm × 2 cm Opta-5 balloon at 10 atm. The residual stenosis was 0% (Figure 27.2).

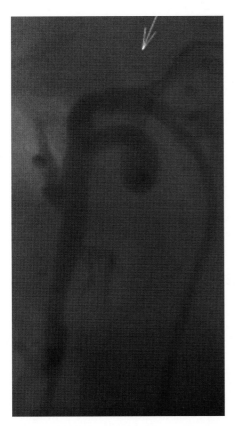

Figure 27.2 *Lateral view of the final post-stent dilatation with an excellent result.*

115

Commentary

A high degree of suspicion is necessary when taking a history for mesenteric ischemia. Generally speaking, two of the three vessels (celiac, SMA or inferior mesenteric artery) must be affected for a patient to be symptomatic, but this is not always the case.

The approach to these vessels is either from above (brachial) or via the femoral artery. The sharp angle from the aorta can occasionally pose a difficult problem when attempting to advance a relatively rigid stent across a stenosis. For this reason, we prefer to use shorter stents ($\leq$ 15 mm) and more flexible stents. Otherwise, the general technique is very similar to that for renal stent placement.

Case 28: Endovascular Management of Traumatic Renal Artery Dissection

James T Lee, Rodney A White

Background

A 22-year-old man was admitted after jumping head first out of a fourth floor window. Injuries sustained included bilateral frontal contusions with associated skull and facial fractures. Gross hematuria was observed on placement of a Foley catheter. Serum chemistry demonstrated a creatinine of 2.0 mg/dl. The initial computed tomography (CT) scan of the abdomen clearly depicts decreased enhancement and delayed excretion of the right kidney, indicating diminished overall perfusion (Figure 28.1). A small fracture is also noted. There was no evidence of a perinephric hematoma, retroperitoneal hemorrhage or free fluid in the abdomen.

Procedure

The angiographic examination with selective renal artery catheterization demonstrated two areas of intimal injury of the right renal artery (Figure 28.2).

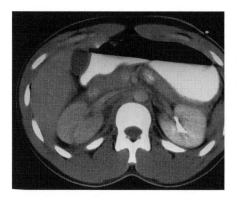

Figure 28.1 *Intravenous enhanced computed tomography of the abdomen before stent placement.*

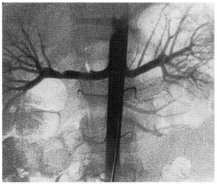

Figure 28.2 *Selective renal arteriogram illustrating the intimal flaps that narrow the lumen of the extrahilar right renal artery.*

Disruption of the intima is seen at approximately 0.5 cm and at 3.0 cm from the orifice of the right renal artery. Although narrowing of the vessel lumen is evident on oblique views, distal perfusion is present. No evidence of peripheral infarction, extravasation of contrast or thrombus was identified. The remainder of the aortogram demonstrated no other major vessel injury. Two Palmaz stents (P204) were deployed on 5 mm balloons without incident using a guiding catheter (Figure 28.3).

Commentary

Renovascular injuries from blunt trauma occur in 1–4% of patients with renal injury. When it does occur, commonly renal parenchymal injuries prevail. These are often accompanied by surrounding perirenal hematomas and associated visceral trauma which often preclude surgical intervention.

The primary goal of definitive management is to avert the clinical consequences of dissection, which were invariably manifestations resulting in renal ischemia. Among the most common are thrombosis, infarction, progressive oliguria and the development of renovascular hypertension. Standard recommendations for the management of non-occluding intimal injuries in most major branches of the arterial tree include correction of the defect to prevent progression to occlusion. This dictum has classically been accomplished through surgical revascularization, but percutaneous endovascular placement of prosthetic stents has met with success.

Management of traumatic renal artery dissection remains controversial. The encouraging outcome of recent experience supports consideration of endovascular therapy for traumatic renal artery dissection in patients with multiple concomitant acute injuries.

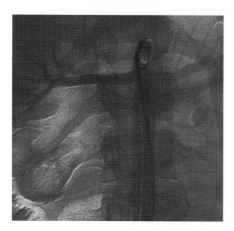

Figure 28.3 *Complete exclusion of the intimal defects with no residual stenosis and normal distal perfusion seen on the final angiogram.*

Acknowledgement

The authors would like to express their gratitude to Gloria Stevens for her timely preparation of the figures for this work.

References

1. Kaufman JL, Charles RD, Dhiraj MS, Leather RP, Renal artery intimal flaps after blunt trauma: Indications for nonoperative therapy. *J Vasc Surg* 1988;**8**:33–7.

2. Whigham CJ Jr, Bodenhamer JR, Miller JK, Use of the Palmaz stent in primary treatment of renal artery intimal injury secondary to blunt trauma. *J Vasc Interv Radiol* 1995;**6**:175–8.

3. Goodman D, Saibil EA, Kodama RT, Traumatic intimal tear of the renal artery treated by insertion of a Palmaz stent. *Cardiovasc Interv Radiol* 1998;**21**:69–72.

Case 29: Renal stent for pulmonary edema/congestive heart failure

Christoph Kalka, Kenneth Rosenfield

Background

A 69-year-old white woman with a 10-year history of hypertension presented in pulmonary edema secondary to florid congestive heart failure (CHF). Examination revealed a blood pressure of 220/160 mmHg and serum creatinine levels increased to 8 mg/dl from a previous baseline of 1.4 mg/dl. Hemodialysis was initiated because of the loss of excretory function and for fluid and electrolyte management.

Ischemic nephropathy was suspected in this patient presenting with acute renal failure, with no signs of acute tubular necrosis or other renal disease. Renal scanning and fractional flow assessment with [^{99m}Tc]mertiatide (MAG-3) showed decreased uptake of the tracer in the right kidney and progressive accumulation in the left kidney without definite evidence of tracer excretion.

Procedure

An abdominal angiogram confirmed a small right renal artery with a subtotal occlusion, supplying a very small kidney. The left renal artery was occluded with a very small 'nubbin' corresponding to the origin of that occluded vessel (Figure 29.1). The left renal artery was recanalized with a guidewire (Figure 29.2), and

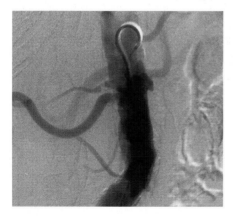

Figure 29.1 *Baseline arteriogram showing a small right renal artery with a subtotal occlusion. The left renal artery is occluded at the ostium without visualization of the distal artery on a nephrogram. There is a small 'nubbin' corresponding to the origin of the occluded vessel.*

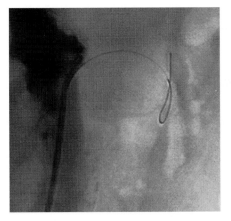

Figure 29.2 *Recanalization of the occluded left renal artery with a guidewire.*

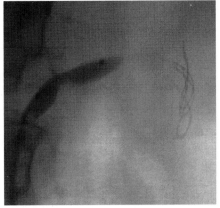

Figure 29.3 *Balloon angioplasty of recanalized left renal artery.*

then balloon angioplasty was performed (Figure 29.3). A Corinthian IQ stent was deployed (Figure 29.4). She received two stents.

Commentary

The diagnostic work-up indicated a single functioning kidney with an occluded renal artery. The images show an ostial occlusion of the left renal artery without visualization of the distal artery on a nephrogram (see Figure 29.1). The role of renal vascular disease in contributing to the progression of renal failure is an important clinical problem that can be expected to increase in incidence and prevalence as the ageing population at risk for atherosclerotic complications grows. Some investigators have estimated that 25% of the patients aged over 60 years presenting with end-stage renal disease (ESRD) have atherosclerotic renovascular disease as a cause of renal failure.

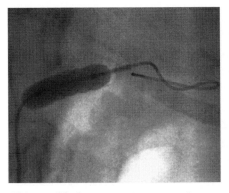

Figure 29.4 *Stent deployment with an 18-mm-long Corinthian IQ stent.*

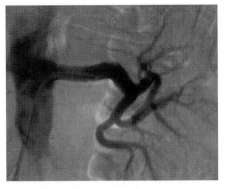

Figure 29.5 *Final arteriogram with complete recanalization of the left renal artery.*

Percutaneous revascularization of renal artery stenosis (RAS) for preservation of renal function involves conventional balloon angioplasty, with or without stenting. Guiding catheter techniques are commonly employed, which involve the use of peripheral guidewires and balloon catheters. The introduction of stents in conjunction with angioplasty has overcome technical problems such as inadequate dilatation, potential for dissection, elastic recoil or high re-stenosis rate.

In the case presented, renal function was completely lost with fluid overload and secondary CHF with pulmonary edema. A significant rise in the serum creatinine and assymetry of the kidney size suggested a single functional kidney with a hemodynamically significant RAS. Reasons for the acute decompensation of the renal function are a spontaneous progression of RAS to occlusion or, in this case more probably, an acute thrombotic occlusion of a severely stenotic RAS.

Restoration of normal function was achieved by balloon angioplasty and stenting of the occluded renal artery. The patient's urine output increased shortly after the intervention and she was free of dialysis within 2 days of the procedure. Her serum creatinine dropped to 1.8 mg/dl and remained high–normal at a 1-month follow-up.

Further studies are needed to address the issue of ischemic nephropathy to determine which patients will benefit and when to intervene.

References

1. Mailloux LU, Napolitano B, Belluci AG et al, Renal vascular disease causing end-stage renal disease, incidence, clinical correlates, and outcomes. *Am J Kidney Dis* 1994;**24**:622–9.

2. Dejani H, Eisen TD, Finkelstein FO, Revascularization of renal artery stenosis in patients with renal insufficiency. *Am J Kidney Dis* 2000;**36**:752–8.

3. Tuttle KR, Chouinard RF, Webber JT et al, Treatment of atherosclerotic ostial renal artery stenosis with the intravascular stent. *Am J Kidney Dis* 1998;32:611–22.

4. Paulsen D, Kløw N-E, Rogstad B et al, Preservation of renal function by percutaneous transluminal angioplasty in ischemic renal disease. *Nephrol Dial Transplant* 1999;**14**:1454–61.

5. Watson PS, Hadjipetrou P, Cox SV et al, Effect of renal artery stenting on renal function and size in patients with atherosclerotic renovascular disease. *Circulation* 2000;**102**:1671–7.

6. Novick AC, Textor SC, Bodie B, Khauli RB, Revascularization to preserve renal function in patients with atherosclerotic renovascular disease. *Urol Clin North Am* 1984;11:477–90.

7. Harden PN, MacLeod MJ, Rodger RSC, Effect of renal-artery stenting on progression of renovascular renal failure. *Lancet* 1997;**349**:1133–6.

CASE 30: RENAL ARTERY FIBROMUSCULAR DYSPLASIA: DIAGNOSIS AND TREATMENT

Manohar Gowda, Audrey Loeb, Paul Kramer

Background

A 47-year-old woman sustained a stroke when her systolic blood pressure was 235 mmHg and was evaluated because of increasing difficulty controlling her hypertension. She was screened for renal artery stenosis with color-flow duplex imaging (CFDI), which suggested right renal artery stenosis.

Procedure

Renal arteriography showed a normal left renal artery. The right renal artery was slightly narrowed in its distal two-thirds, and the luminal edge had a slightly scalloped appearance (Figure 30.1). Intravascular ultrasonography (IVUS) indicated fluttering membranes and crescentic ridges throughout the middle and distal segments of the right renal artery (Figure 30.2). The classic beaded appearance of fibromuscular dysplasia (FMD) was not present.

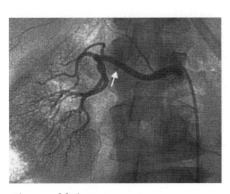

Figure 30.1 *Right renal artery arteriogram (pre-angioplasty).*

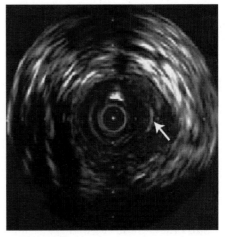

Figure 30.2 *Intravascular ultrasound (pre-angioplasty).*

Angioplasty was performed with a non-compliant 5 mm × 4 cm balloon (Ultra-Thin Diamond: Boston Scientific Corp., Natick, MA, USA) inflated to a pressure of 12 atm in the middle and distal segments of the right renal artery. On fluoroscopy, the balloon appeared to be fully expanded and appropriately slightly oversized in comparison with the proximal reference segment (Figure 30.3). IVUS after this balloon inflation showed persistence of essentially all of the defects seen at baseline throughout the middle and distal segments (Figure 30.4), with no apparent change in the angiographic appearance (Figure 30.5). Repeat balloon dilatation was performed using the same balloon inflated to 15 atm. The fluoroscopic appearance of the balloon was the same as at 12 atm (Figure 30.6). Repeat IVUS of the middle and distal segments now showed a markedly improved lumen diameter and elimination of the fluttering

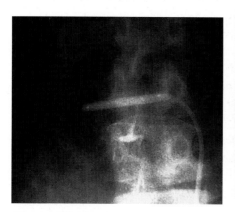

Figure 30.3 *Right renal artery balloon angioplasty 12 atm.*

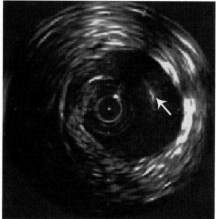

Figure 30.4 *Right renal artery intravascular ultrasonography after balloon angioplasty at 12 atm.*

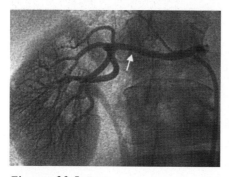

Figure 30.5 *Right renal artery arteriogram after balloon angioplasty at 12 atm.*

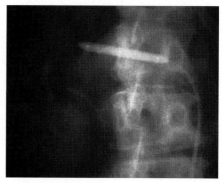

Figure 30.6 *Right renal artery balloon angioplasty at 15 atm.*

124

membranous defects seen at baseline (Figure 30.7), and final arteriography showed improved diameter and smoothed lumen appearance in the treated segments (Figure 30.8).

Commentary

Fibromuscular dysplasia represents the second most common cause of renal artery stenosis (RAS). It occurs earlier in life than atherosclerotic RAS, affects women up to eight times more commonly than men, and generally spares the proximal renal segment, typically being localized in the middle and distal segments and occasionally extending into primary branches.

Non-invasive screening with CFDI can reveal the flow disturbances associated with RAS and suggests the diagnosis of FMD when they occur beyond the proximal segment, this being the typical site of atherosclerotic obstruction. Abnormal CFDI findings include high-flow velocity, high-flow velocity ratio relative to adjacent aortic flow velocity, and abnormal, non-laminar flow patterns (such as aliasing and spiralling flow).

The classic arteriographic finding in FMD is a beaded appearance produced by multiple, eccentric, cleft-like stenoses appearing beyond the most proximal segment of the renal artery. However, patients identified with flow abnormalities with CFDI may have arteriograms, which are entirely normal, or may show mild luminal narrowing or irregularity as seen in this case. IVUS can depict endoluminal and arterial wall anatomy which can be underestimated or even completely inapparent on arteriography. In FMD, IVUS can demonstrate

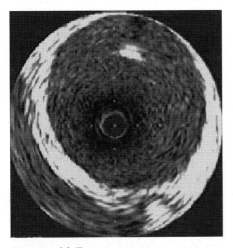

Figure 30.7 *Right renal artery intravascular ultrasonography after balloon angioplasty at 15 atm.*

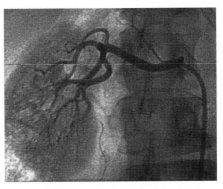

Figure 30.8 *Right renal artery arteriogram after balloon angioplasty at 15 atm.*

125

endoluminal abnormalities including: discrete, fixed, eccentric ridges; fluttering membranes; and/or spiralling longitudinal folds.

This case demonstrates the supplementary role of IVUS in confirming the presence of obstructive renal artery FMD even when the arteriogram does not convincingly indicate the diagnosis. Further, this case demonstrates that very high balloon inflation pressures may be required to obliterate the obstructive elements characteristic of FMD, even when balloon sizing appears appropriate and inflation at lower pressures appears to result in complete balloon expansion.

References

1. King BF Jr, Diagnostic imaging evaluation of renovascular hypertension. *Abdom Imaging* 1995;**20**:395–405.

2. Luscher TF, Lie JT, Stanson AW, Arterial fibromuscular dysplasia. *Mayo Clin Proc* 1987;**62**:931–52.

3. Tegtmeyer CJ, Elson J, Glass TA, Percutaneous transluminal angioplasty: the treatment of choice for renovascular hypertension due to fibromuscular dysplasia. *Radiology* 1982;**143**:631–7.

CASE 31: PROTECTED RENAL ANGIOPLASTY

Michel Henry, Isabelle Henry

Background

Percutaneous transluminal angioplasty techniques have become the cornerstone of therapeutic strategy for renal artery stenosis. Occasionally, even after successful technical results, a decline in renal function may be noted in a subset of patients. Recently, Isles et al[2] published a review of 10 studies, including 416 stent placement procedures in 379 patients treated for renal artery stenosis. Although technical success was high (96–100%), renal function improved in 26%, stabilized in 48% and deteriorated in 26% of the patients.

Potential reasons for deterioration of renal function after angioplasty and stenting include contrast nephrotoxicity, return of high pressure perfusion to a previously hypoperfused glomerular bed and progression of pre-existing renal disease although microembolization to the renal parenchyma has a significant role. This is caused by the release of microscopic plaque fragments and cholesterol crystals from the renal artery lesion or the aorta into parenchyme renal vasculature during the procedure.

The long-term impact of renal embolization is suggested by a study in which renal biopsy was performed during surgery for renal artery stenosis. In this study, 36% of patients had biopsy-proven atheroemboli after renal bypass surgery, and atheroembolic renal disease correlated significantly with decreased patient survival. Of those patients with atheroemboli there was a decreased 5-year survival rate of 54% versus 85% in those patients without emboli.

To eliminate the risk of atheroembolic material being flushed into the renal parenchyma, we applied a novel technique of balloon angioplasty and stenting

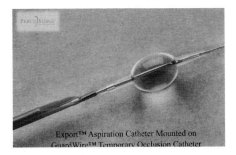

Figure 31.1 Export™ aspiration catheter mounted on GuardWire™ occlusion catheter

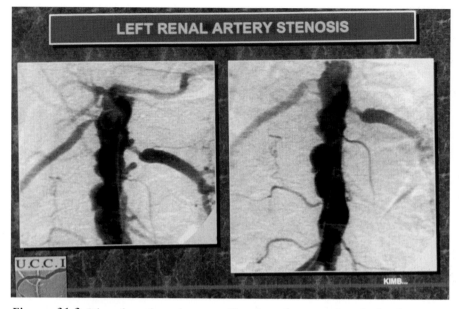

Figure 31.2 Bilateral renal ostial stenosis. Very diseased aorta with multiple atheromatous plaques

with distal protection using the PercuSurge Guardwire (Medtronic, Minneapolis, MN, USA), a concept currently being used in aortocoronary saphenous vein graft re-stenosis and carotid artery angioplasty (Figure 31.1).

A 59-year-old patient with a past history of both coronary and carotid angioplasty now presents with severe hypertension (220/120 mmHg). Baseline angiography revealed a tight left ostial renal artery stenosis and the abdominal aorta was very diseased with multiple atheromatous plaques (Figure 31.2). The baseline serum creatinine was 1.3 mg/dl.

Procedure

Femoral arterial access with a 8 Fr sheath was obtained. A 8 Fr renal, double-curve, guiding catheter was placed at the ostium of the left renal artery. The Guardwire was advanced across the lesion. The distal occlusion ballon was inflated (Figure 31.3). The ostial lesion was predilated with a 6 mm balloon (Speedy Bypass: Boston Scientific Corp., Watertown, MA). A Palmaz 154 stent (Cordis, Miami, FL) was deployed with the 6 mm angioplasty balloon (Figure 31.3). The balloon catheter was exchanged for the aspiration Export catheter and visible debris was removed (Figure 31.4). The distal balloon was then deflated after an occlusion time of 13 min. Final angiography revealed an excellent result (see Figure 31.3). The 6-month follow-up revealed the blood pressure to be 160/90 mmHg and the serum creatinine was 1.2 mg/dl.

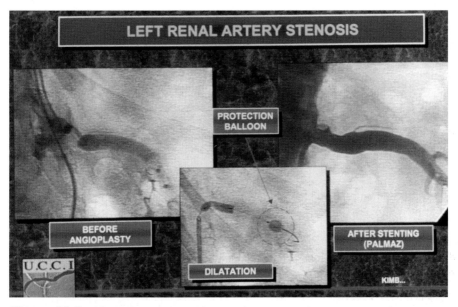

Figure 31.3 *Left renal artery angioplasty and stenting under protection with Percusurge GuardWire*

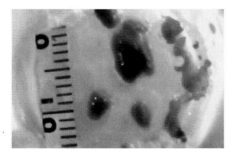

Figure 31.4 *Aspirated debris with aspiration catheter*

Commentary

We have used this technique in 35 atherosclerotic renal arterial stenoses in 30 patients. All were hypertensive, ten with moderate and two with severe renal dysfunction. The immediate technical success was 100%. Visible debris was aspirated from all patients. The mean particle number was 98.1±60 per procedure (13–208), and diameter 201.2±76.0 μm (38–6206 μm) (Figure 31.5). The mean renal artery occlusion time was 6.55±2.46 min. At a mean follow-up of 6.7±2.9 months, creatinine levels dropped from 1.34±3.5 mg/dl to 1.24±0.31 mg/dl. At the 6-month follow-up we observed no renal function deterioration in any patient. Five patients with baseline renal insufficiency had improved after the procedure. Systolic and diastolic blood pressures dropped from 167±15.2 mmHg to 154.7±12.3 mmHg and 103±12 mmHg to 93.2±6.8 mmHg after the procedure, respectively.

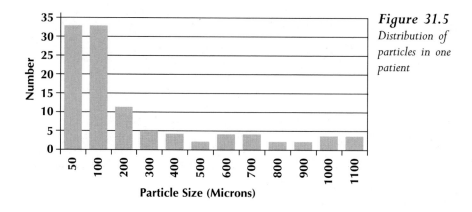

Figure 31.5
Distribution of particles in one patient

Protection against atheroembolism of the renal parenchyma is feasible. Who therefore needs protection during renal angioplasty and stenting? Today, patients who may benefit most are those with severe atheroaortic disease, ostial renal stenosis, severely calcific or thrombotic lesions and, of great importance in our opinion, patients with either a solitary kidney or already impaired renal function.

References

1. Henry M, Amor M, Henry I et al, Stent placement in the renal artery: three-year experience with the Palmaz stent. *J Endovasc Surg* 1999;**6**:42–51.

2. Isles CG, Robertson S, Hill D, Management of renovascular disease: a review of renal artery stenting in ten studies. *Q J Med* 1999;**92**:159–67.

3. Scolari F, Bracchi M, Valzorio B et al, Cholesterol atheromatous embolism: an increasingly recognized cause of acute renal failure. *Nephrol Dial Transplant* 1996;**11**:1607–12.

4. Saleem S, Lakkis FG, Martinez-Maldonado M, Atheroembolic renal disease. *Semin Nephrol* 1996;**16**:309–18.

5. Krishnamurthi V, Novick AC, Myles JL, Atheroembolic renal disease: effect on morbidity and survival after revascularization for atherosclerotic renal artery stenosis. *J Urol* 1999;**161**:1093–6.

6. Thadhani RI, Camargo CA Jr, Xavier RJ et al, Atheroembolic renal failure after invasive procedures. Natural history based on 52 histologically proven cases. *Medicine (Baltimore)* 1995;**74**:350–8.

7. Henry M, Amor M, Henry I et al, Carotid stenting with cerebral protection. First clinical experience using the PercuSurge Guardwire system. *J Endovasc Surg* 1999;**6**:321–31.

CASE 32: FIBROMUSCULAR DYSPLASIA CAUSING RENOVASCULAR HYPERTENSION: HEMODYNAMIC LESION ASSESSMENT

Gary M Ansel

Background

A 36-year-old woman with progressively worsening hypertension was referred for evaluation. She was initially diagnosed 7 years ago, and over the past several months, the hypotension had become increasingly difficult to control with multiple medications.

Procedure

A non-selective aortogram was obtained with a 6 Fr pigtail catheter injecting 12 ml/s for 3 s of non-ionic contrast. It demonstrated unilateral fibromuscular dysplasia (FMD) of the right kidney (Figure 32.1). Assessing the severity of these lesions has traditionally been very difficult because the severity of the stenosis is not clearly seen. A 0.014-inch pressure wire (RADI) was advanced across the lesion and a 45 mmHg gradient was measured with the guiding catheter in the aorta (Figure 32.2). Using a 6 Fr sheath as a guiding catheter, a 6 mm × 2 cm balloon was inflated in the right renal artery (Figure 32.3). The post-percutaneous transluminal angioplasty angiogram demonstrated an excellent result and the residual pressure gradient was less than 10 mmHg (Figure 32.4).

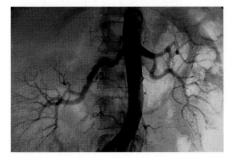

Figure 32.1 *Abdominal aortogram demonstrating fibromuscular dysplasia of the left renal artery.*

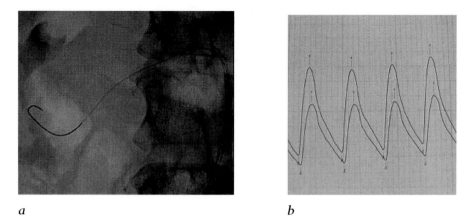

a

b

Figure 32.2 (a) Pressure wire in left renal artery. (b) Pre-angioplasty pressure gradient.

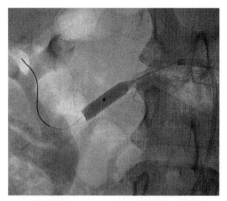

Figure 32.3 Balloon angioplasty of right renal artery.

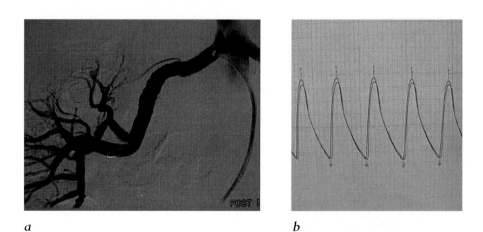

a

b

Figure 32.4 (a) Post-angioplasty angiogram. (b) Post-angioplasty pressure wire measurements showing resolution of gradient.

132

Commentary

This case illustrates the treatment of FMD as a cause of renovascular hypertension. In general, these lesions are well treated with balloon angioplasty alone. The assessment of the angiographic lesion is very difficult. The use of the 0.014-inch pressure wire helps to assess the severity of the lesion and confirm that an adequate angioplasty result has been obtained.

CASE 33: RENAL INTERVENTION FOR NEW-ONSET RENAL FAILURE

Gary M Ansel

Background

A 73-year-old woman with symptomatic peripheral vascular disease, severe hypertension and new-onset dialysis for 2 weeks presented with decompensated congestive heart failure. On renal ultrasonography, her left kidney was 9.2 cm and her right kidney was 10.4 cm in length.

Procedure

An abdominal aortogram demonstrated bilateral critical renal artery stenosis (Figure 33.1). As a result of the cephalad orientation of the renal ostia, an upper extremity approach was chosen. While gaining access, a severe asymptomatic left subclavian stenosis was encountered which made catheter manipulation difficult. For this reason it was treated with stent implantation (Figure 33.2). A 6 Fr 90-cm-long sheath with a multipurpose catheter as an introducer was advanced to the renal arteries. Bilateral balloon-expandable stents were deployed over a 0.035-inch guidewire (Figures 33.3 and 33.4).

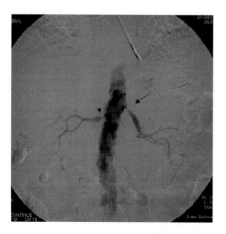

Figure 33.1 *Abdominal angiogram showing severe bilateral renal artery stenosis (arrows), down-going renal vessels and a shaggy aorta.*

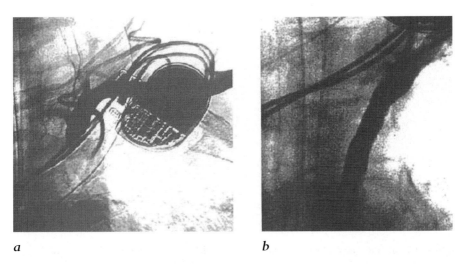

a   b

Figure 33.2 (a) Angiogram demonstrating left subclavian stenosis. (b) Subclavian artery after balloon-expandable stent placement.

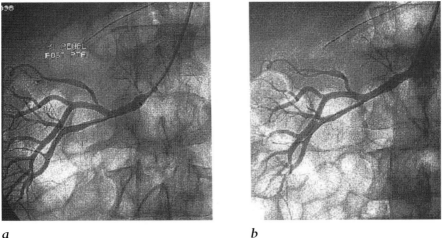

a   b

Figure 33.3 (a) Selective right renal angiogram. (b) Post-balloon-expandable stent placement.

The patient immediately improved, with her creatinine level falling to 1.9 mg/dl at 48 hours and she no longer required hemodialysis. Her blood pressure was controlled on two medications and she has had no recurrent admissions for congestive heart failure.

Commentary

This case illustrates several important points. First, all patients with new-onset renal failure and evidence of atherosclerosis elsewhere should be evaluated for

135

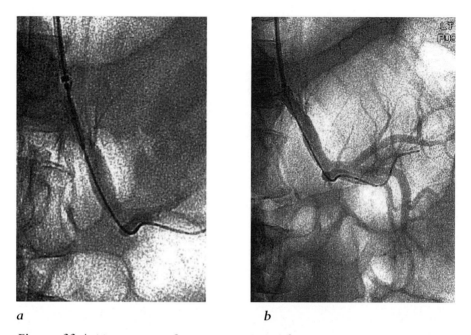

a   b

Figure 33.4 *(a) Angiogram of stent positioning in left renal artery. (b) Post-balloon-expandable stent placement.*

renal vascular disease. Second, after successful treatment of bilateral renal artery disease or a solitary kidney patients should be monitored for post-obstructive diuresis and/or hypotension.

CASE 34: RENAL ARTERY THROMBOEMBOLIZATION AFTER STENT PLACEMENT: SUCCESSFUL TREATMENT WITH COMBINATION GLYCOPROTEIN IIb/IIIa PLATELET RECEPTOR ANTAGONISTS AND LYTIC THERAPY

Gary M Ansel

Background

A 73-year-old woman with chronic renal insufficiency (creatinine > 2.0 mg/dl for 2 years) presented for evaluation with accelerated hypertension on four antihypertensive medications, and worsening of her renal failure with a serum creatinine of 2.9 mg/dl.

Procedure

The baseline aortogram (Figure 34.1) demonstrates bilateral renal artery stenosis (arrows) with absent celiac and superior mesenteric arteries. A selective right

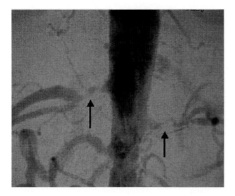

Figure 34.1 *Abdominal aortic angiogram showing bilateral proximal renal artery stenoses (arrows).*

renal angiogram performed with a 6 Fr internal mammary artery (IMA) catheter demonstrates severe proximal stenosis. Using a 7 Fr guiding catheter, the lesion is crossed with an 0.014-inch guidewire (upper branch). Primary stent placement with a 5-mm stent was performed (Figure 34.2). During deployment, the patient complained of severe back pain which was persistent. Her blood pressure elevated to 220/110 mmHg. The post-stent deployment angiogram demonstrates evidence of distal thromboembolism and occlusion of the major inferior branch (Figure 34.3).

Several options were considered. One option would include an intra-arterial infusion of a lytic agent, but this was not chosen because it would probably take more than 4 hours, and rapid reperfusion is essential if kidney salvage is the goal. The second choice was mechanical thrombectomy (Possis AngioJet) but this was not chosen because the emboli were diffuse and very distal in the small branches. Surgical embolectomy was not considered to be a reasonable option. Finally, the decision was made to use a combination of intravenous abciximab (Reopro: Lily, Indianapolis, IN, USA) given in the standard coronary dose

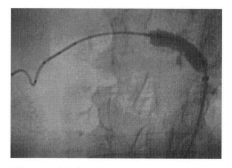

Figure 34.2 Primary balloon-expandable stent placement in the right renal artery.

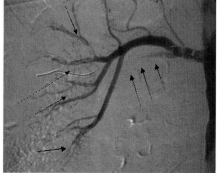

Figure 34.3 Post-stent angiogram with diffuse thromboembolization and loss of the inferior branch.

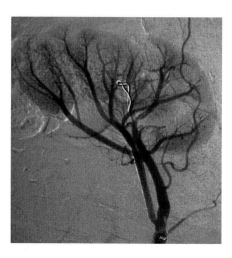

Figure 34.4 Repeat angiogram after standard intravenous abciximab bolus and 7 mg tissue plasminogen activator into the renal artery over 30 min. Note the resolution of thrombus and reconstitution of the inferior branch vessel.

(0.25 mg/kg bolus) and a 30-min tissue plasminogen activator (rtPTA) infusion of 7 mg. Re-look angiography demonstrated dramatic improvement in flow and resolution of distal emboli (Figure 34.4). The patient's back pain resolved. The left renal stent procedure was competed uneventfully. At 24 hours her serum creatinine was 2.6 mg/dl, and at 48 hours it had dropped to 2.1 mg/dl. Her blood pressure was 140/85 mmHg on only one medication.

Commentary

This patient developed an unusual but catastrophic complication of renal artery intervention – distal thromboembolization. The decision to treat the patient with a combination of a glycoprotein IIb/IIIa platelet inhibitor and a selective infusion of a thrombolytic agent has not been described in this situation. However, given the positive results of several acute myocardial infarction trials using combined therapy, it seemed to be a reasonable option in this instance. In the future, the use of devices that protect against emboli may make this complication less likely; however, in this patient, with the proximal bifurcation of her renal artery, it would not have been an option.

IV AORTO-ILIAC AND LOWER EXTREMITY INTERVENTIONS

Case 35: Iliac artery intervention for an atheroembolic lesion

J Michael Bacharach

Background

A 59-year-old woman presented with the sudden onset of blue discoloration of the left great toe. She described antecedent claudication symptoms, but was not severely limited before the sudden discoloration of this toe. Physical examination demonstrated marked bluish discoloration of the left great toe with ischemic changes. Pulse examination demonstrated palpable femoral, popliteal and posterior tibial pulses bilaterally.

Non-invasive vascular studies with segmental pressures and Doppler waveforms demonstrated a thigh index that was mildly reduced at 0.8 and a left ankle brachial index (ABI) of 0.8. The right ABI was normal.

Procedure

Abdominal aortography demonstrated a normal appearing aorta and right common iliac artery, with a critical, eccentric, left common iliac stenosis (Figure 35.1). The pelvic arteriogram highlights the severe focal lesion involving the left common iliac artery in its midportion (Figure 35.2). Further angiographic assessment of the infrainguinal portion of the left leg demonstrated occlusion of the distal anterior tibial artery (Figure 35.3).

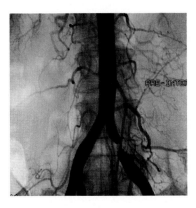

Figure 35.1 *Aortogram demonstrating normal aorta and right iliac artery with a critical narrowing of the left common iliac artery.*

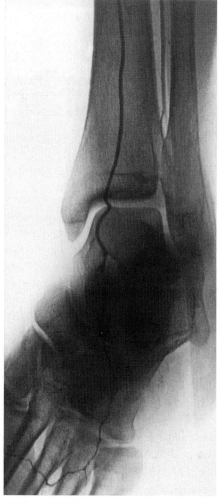

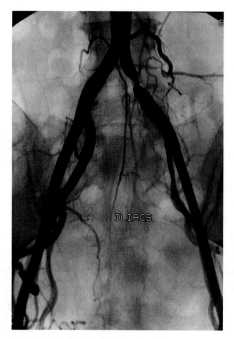

Figure 35.2 *Pelvic arteriogram demonstrating the high-grade lesion of the left iliac artery with post-stenotic dilatation.*

Figure 35.3 *Distal run-off angiogram demonstrating occlusion (cut-off) of the anterior tibial artery at the ankle.*

Using a 7 Fr crossover sheath (Balkan: Cook Inc., Bloomington, IN, USA), the lesion was crossed in an anterograde fashion with a steerable 0.035-inch guidewire. Balloon pre-dilatation was performed and a 12 mm × 40 mm self-expanding SMART (Cordis, Miami, FL) stent was deployed (Figure 35.4). The post-stent angiogram demonstrated a widely patent lumen (Figure 35.5).

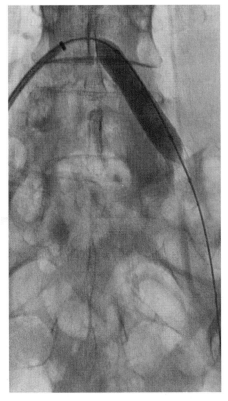

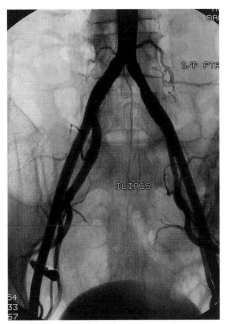

Figure 35.4 *Balloon angioplasty pre-dilatation.*

Figure 35.5 *Final angiogram after SMART stent deployment.*

Commentary

The clinical and angiographic data suggest a focal iliac lesion that has embolized, causing the ischemic changes to the left great toe. Angiographically there was no evidence of multilevel arterial occlusive disease. The left iliac artery lesion was focal and amenable to endovascular repair.

Currently there are very few data to support the use of balloon angioplasty and stenting for focal embolic lesions, although anecdotally numerous investigators have described an endovascular approach to focal lesions.

In this particular case, we felt that an endovascular approach using a self-expanding stent from the contralateral side would be a reasonable choice. A self-expanding stent was chosen because of its closer cell design, as well as the ability to adapt and conform to the arterial morphology, noting the post-stenotic dilatation just beyond the high-grade lesion. It was felt that this would reduce the likelihood of iliac artery dissection and the potential need for multiple stents. Clinically the patient improved dramatically and subsequently the ischemic changes of the left great toe resolved.

145

Case 36: Distal Aortoiliac Intervention

J Michael Bacharach

Background

A 46-year-old white man presents with a 5-year history of progressively worsening, lower extremity claudication. He is now unable to perform his usual daily activities. Physical examination revealed a robust man, 6 foot (1.8 m), and 260 pounds (120 kg). He was obese, with normal blood pressure in both arms and no palpable pulses in either lower extremity. Non-invasive studies revealed an ankle brachial index (ABI) of 0.87 and 0.68 for the right and left legs, respectively.

Procedure

Abdominal aortography performed via brachial artery access demonstrated occlusion of the distal aorta with extensive lumbar collateral vessels (Figure 36.1). Late phase filling demonstrates reconstitution of the external iliac arteries via collaterals from the lumbar and the internal iliac arteries (Figure 36.2).

Access was gained in the right common femoral artery with a long 7 Fr sheath and a 0.035-inch glidewire (Terumo: Boston Scientific Corp., Watertown, MA, USA) was used to cross the right iliac occlusion. A 6 Fr multipurpose

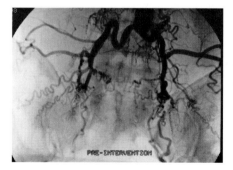

Figure 36.1 *Pelvic arteriogram demonstrating occlusion of the terminal aorta with extensive lumbar artery collaterals.*

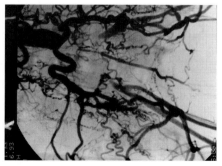

Figure 36.2 *Pelvic arteriogram (late phase) demonstrating reconstitution of bilateral external iliac arteries.*

catheter was advanced over the glidewire into the aorta and contrast was injected to confirm the intraluminal location of the wire.

The left common femoral artery was entered and a long 7 Fr sheath inserted. The left iliac occlusion was crossed with an 0.035-inch angled glidewire, and the intraluminal position of the wire was confirmed with contrast injections. 'Kissing' balloon angioplasty was carried out with 8 mm × 4 cm Opta-5 (Cordis, Miami, FL) balloons. The long 7 Fr sheaths were then advanced into the terminal aorta and two Palmaz 394 balloon-expandable stents (Cordis) were mounted on the percutaneous transluminal angioplasty balloons, and deployed with a 'kissing' balloon inflation in the terminal aorta and proximal common iliac artery. Two additional Palmaz 394 stents were placed contiguous with the initial stents in the common iliac arteries using the 8-mm balloons. Post-intervention demonstrates recanalization with stenting of the aortic bifurcation and proximal iliac arteries (Figure 36.3).

Commentary

The patient was young, with severe functional limitation secondary to claudication. The angiogram demonstrated occlusion of the distal aorta. The extensive collaterals suggested that this was a chronic, rather than an acute, occlusion and is consistent with the patient's 5-year history of claudication symptoms.

In the past, the standard recommendation for this case would have been aortoiliac or aortobifemoral bypass surgery. The current case offers an alternative to surgical revascularization. There is concern about preserving sexual function and about the morbidity and mortality of surgery balanced against the durability or patency of iliac intervention.

This case highlights the use of endovascular stents for reconstruction of total occlusions of the aortoiliac segment. Although the primary patency is slightly lower for balloon angioplasty alone in occlusions compared with a surgical approach, there appears to be little difference between the two techniques when stents are deployed.

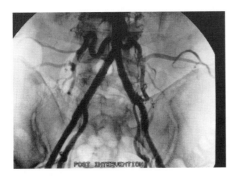

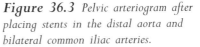

Figure 36.3 *Pelvic arteriogram after placing stents in the distal aorta and bilateral common iliac arteries.*

References

1. DeVries SO, Hunink MG, Results of aortic bifurcation grafts for aortoiliac occlusive disease: A meta-analysis. *J Vasc Surg* 1997;**26**:558–69.

2. Bosch JL, Hunink MG, Meta-analysis of the results of percutaneous transluminal angioplasty and stent placement for aorto-iliac occlusive disease. *Radiology* 1997;**204**:87–96.

3. Scheinert D, Schroder M, Balzer JO et al, Stent-supported reconstruction of the aorto-iliac bifurcation with the kissing technique. *Circulation* 1999;**100**(suppl 19):II295–300.

Case 37: Infrarenal Aortic Stenting to Relieve Disabling Claudication

Bahij N Khuri, Fadi Naddour, D Luke Glancy

Background

A 57-year-old woman presented with an 8-month history of claudication of the hips, buttocks and thighs on walking less than a two blocks (Fontaine IIb). Physical examination revealed abdominal bruits with diminished femoral pulses and an ankle brachial index (ABI) of 0.7 in both legs at rest.

Procedure

A 8 Fr 35-cm-long femoral sheath (Brite-Tip: Cordis, Miami, FL, USA) was inserted and advanced over a 175-cm, 0.035-inch Wholey wire (Mallinckrodt, St Louis, MO). With contrast material injected through the sheath, an aortogram was obtained in the arteroposterior and lateral projections (Figures 37.1 and 37.2). A systolic pressure gradient of 40 mmHg was recorded on catheter pullback across the abdominal aortic stenosis. Heparin 5000 IU was given intravenously, and the activated clotting time was maintained above 250 s. A 6.2 Fr, 20-MHz Sonicath (Boston Scientific Corp., Watertown, MA) intravascular

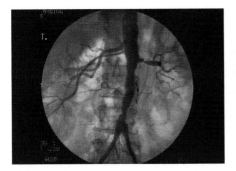

Figure 37.1 *Abdominal aortogram in the anteroposterior projection, showing critical stenoses in the left renal artery and the distal infrarenal aorta.*

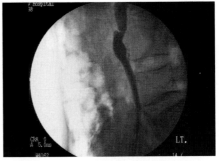

Figure 37.2 *Abdominal aortogram in the lateral projection, showing the eccentric nature of the plaque.*

ultrasonography catheter was used to image the infrarenal aorta (Figure 37.3).

A P308 Palmaz stent (Cordis, Miami, FL) was crimped by hand onto a 9 mm × 4 cm Powerflex (Cordis) balloon catheter. Direct stenting with this undersized balloon was performed at 10 atm. Serial intravascular ultrasound images guided subsequent stent expansion. The final balloon was a 12 mm × 2 cm Opta LP (Cordis). The final intravascular ultrasonic image (Figure 37.4) and aortogram (Figure 37.5) confirmed an excellent result, and there was no pressure gradient across the stent.

Protamine sulfate was given to reverse anticoagulation. Hemostasis was achieved with hand pressure. The post-procedure ABI was 0.92 bilaterally. After 23 hours of observation, the patient was discharged on 325 mg aspirin/day.

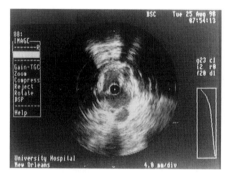

Figure 37.3 *Intravascular ultrasonic image at the lesion site reveals narrowing by eccentric heterogeneous plaque, with shadowing suggestive of deep calcification.*

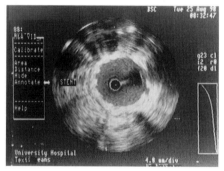

Figure 37.4 *Intravascular ultrasonic image shows resolution of the stenosis and good stent apposition.*

Figure 37.5 *Final aortogram demonstrates resolution of the stenosis without extravasation or dissection.*

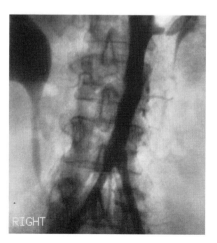

150

Commentary

Balloon dilatation with stent placement has largely replaced open surgical techniques because of its many advantages: no general anesthesia, no abdominal incision, shorter hospital stay, lower morbidity and mortality rates, no nerve damage leading to sexual dysfunction and/or defective anal sphincter tone, and less risk of spinal cord ischemia.[1,2] Infrarenal aortic stenting in the reported literature reveals almost 100% technical success, a 9% complication rate, 92% primary patency and 98% secondary patency at follow-ups of up to 46 months.[1-3] The following are some of the clinical and technical considerations in infrarenal aortic stenting:

1. Clinically important infrarenal aortic stenoses are associated with a resting systolic gradient of ≥ 5 mmHg and/or cause a decrease in femoral arterial pressure of $\geq 15\%$ after flow augmentation by either reactive hyperemia or intra-arterial vasodilators.[4]

2. Angiographic assessment of the celiac, superior and inferior mesenteric arteries is important before aortic intervention is performed, to avoid bowel ischemia if blood flow to the gut is threatened by the stenting procedure. This is particularly important in patients who have undergone a prior surgical procedure that may have compromised mesenteric collateral circulation.

3. The use of a long sheath is advisable to protect the balloon-mounted stent from getting trapped inside the lesion or becoming dislodged from the balloon. After initial deployment of the stent, the sheath is replaced across the lesion to facilitate re-crossing by the ultrasonographic catheter and the final dilatation balloon.

4. Appropriate sizing of the stent is the key to a successful procedure without complications.[5,6] Aortic stenting should be guided by intravascular ultrasonography or quantitative angiography. A patient's complaint of low back pain during balloon inflation may be a warning sign of adventitial stretch, which may occur before aortic rupture.

References

1. Nyman U, Uher P, Lidh M, Lindblad B, Ivancev K, Primary stenting in infrarenal aortic occlusive disease. *Cardiovasc Intervent Radiol* 2000;**23**:97–108.

2. Westcott MA, Bonn J, Comparison of conventional angioplasty with Palmaz stent in the treatment of abdominal aortic stenoses from the STAR registry. *J Vasc Interv Radiol* 1998;**9**:225–31.

3. Long AL, Gaux JC, Raynaud AC et al, Infrarenal aortic stents: Initial clinical experience and angiographic follow-up. *Cardiovasc Intervent Radiol* 1993;**16**:203–8.

151

4. Brewster DC, Clinical and anatomical considerations for surgery in aortoiliac disease and results of surgical treatment. *Circulation* 1991;**83**(suppl I):I42–52.

5. Berger T, Sorensen R, Konrad J, Aortic rupture: A complication of transluminal angioplasty. *Am J Radiol* 1986;**146**:373–4.

6. Cutry AF, Whitley D, Patterson RB, Midaortic pseudoaneurysm complicating extensive endovascular stenting of aortic disease. *J Vasc Surg* 1997;**26**:958–62.

Case 38: Aortoiliac bifurcation stent placement

Rajesh M Dave, Sumeet Sachdev,
John J Young, Thomas M Shimshak

Background

A 69-year-old patient presented with symptoms of lifestyle-limiting, bilateral, lower extremity claudication. On examination, the femoral pulses were diminished bilaterally and the dorsalis pedis pulses were unobtainable. During the evaluation of an ischemic cardiomyopathy (ejection fraction 25%), an abdominal aortogram demonstrated bilateral aortoiliac stenoses. The patient was referred for elective percutaneous revascularization.

Procedure

After sterile preparation and pre-medication two 7 Fr Pinnacle R/O (25 cm) (Terumo, Boston Scientific Medi-Tech, Watertown, MA, USA) sheaths were placed in the right and left femoral arteries over 0.035-inch Wholey Hi-Torque Modified J (Mallinckrodt Inc., St Louis, MO) guidewires. A bolus of 5000 U intravenous heparin was administered. An abdominal aortogram was then performed through a 6 Fr pigtail catheter via the right femoral arterial access (40 ml of iodixanol [Visipaque, Nycomed Inc., Princeton, NJ]) at a rate of 20 ml/s and 600 psi). The angiogram demonstrated a focal, eccentric, calcified subtotal stenosis of the right common iliac artery and a tubular, eccentric, subtotal, left common iliac stenosis (Figure 38.1). In addition, there was no apparent occlusive disease of either the external iliac or the common femoral arteries.

Two 5.0 mm × 40 mm Marshall balloons (Boston Scientific Medi-Tech, Watertown, MA) (75-cm shaft length) were introduced from the left and right femoral approach, simultaneous 'kissing' balloon inflations at the aortoiliac bifurcation were performed at 10 atm. Subsequently, two 8.0 mm × 26 mm Bridge stents (Medtronic AVE, Santa Rosa, CA) were simultaneously deployed at each common iliac artery in a 'kissing' fashion, extending each stent into the distal aorta. An additional 8.0 mm × 27 mm MegaLink stent (Guidant, Advanced Cardiovascular Systems, Temecula, CA) was placed in the distal left common iliac artery. The stents were post-dilated with the same 8 mm × 40 mm Marshall balloons using a 'kissing' technique to a maximum of 10 atm. Contrast injections via the side ports

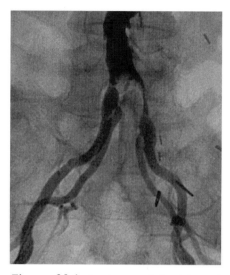

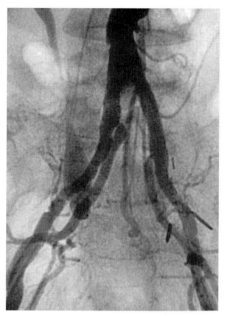

Figure 38.1 *Arteriogram of the abdominal aorta and iliac arteries (anteroposterior projection). 6 Fr pigtail catheter is positioned in the lower abdominal aorta via the right femoral arterial approach. The arteriogram demonstrates focal high-grade disease of both the right and the left common iliac artery ostia. There is also focal non-occlusive disease of the distal right external iliac artery.*

Figure 38.2 *Arteriogram after stenting of the distal aorta and both iliac artery ostia (anteroposterior projection). Simultaneous contrast injection via the side port of 7 Fr long (25 cm) sheaths in each femoral artery demonstrates the wide patency of each common iliac artery. There is focal irregularity of the right external iliac artery.*

of the femoral sheaths (20 ml each) demonstrated patency of the aortoiliac bifurcation and common iliac arteries. There was a localized minor irregularity of the right external iliac artery at the tip of the sheath, which was judged to be insignificant, and no intervention was performed in this area (Figure 38.2). There was no pressure gradient present and the procedure was terminated. The arterial sheaths were removed and manual compression was applied. The patient was discharged from the hospital the following day with an uneventful post-procedure course on aspirin 325 mg/day and clopidogrel 75 mg/day for 30 days.

Routine clinical reassessment was carried out 2 weeks later. At that time, the patient complained of continued bilateral intermittent claudication. In fact, his symptoms were worse than those before the interventional procedure. His physical examination demonstrated diminished femoral pulses and very weak pedal pulses bilaterally. Repeat angiography was recommended.

Repeat aortography was performed via the left femoral approach using a 6 Fr pigtail catheter through a short 6 Fr sheath. This demonstrated wide patency of each common iliac artery. However, there was a lengthy, occlusive dissection, beginning at the proximal portion of the right external iliac artery and extending to the right common femoral artery (Figure 38.3). In addition, the left external iliac artery had mild diffuse tubular narrowing, moderate angulation and a significant stenosis several centimeters proximal to the sheath tip (Figure 38.4). Bilateral external iliac artery angioplasty and stenting were performed. A bolus of 5000 U intravenous heparin was administered.

The left external iliac artery was pre-dilated with a 5 mm × 40 mm Marshall balloon catheter over a 0.035-inch Wholey wire. Several Nitinol SMART stents (Cordis Endovascular, Miami, FL) were then deployed in an overlapping fashion, and post-dilated sequentially with 6.0 mm × 40 mm and 7.0 mm × 40 mm PowerFlex plus balloon catheters (Cordis Endovascular).

The right external iliac artery dissection was crossed with a 0.035-inch Wholey wire and primarily stented with two sequential 7.0 mm × 80 mm and 7.0 mm × 60 mm SMART stents, encompassing the entire external iliac and proximal right common femoral arteries. The external and common femoral artery stents were post-dilated with 7.0 mm × 10 cm and 6.0 mm × 10 cm PowerFlexplus, respectively.

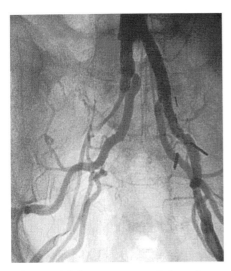

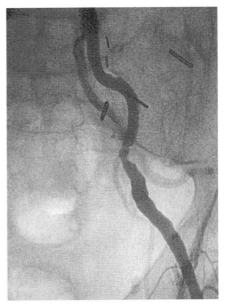

Figure 38.3 *Arteriogram of the right and left iliac arteries (anteroposterior projection). A lengthy subtotal dissection plane is apparent, extending from the proximal portion of the right external iliac artery to the distal segment of the right common femoral artery.*

Figure 38.4 *Left femoral and external iliac arteriogram (anteroposterior projection). A focal stenosis is apparent at the junction of the left external iliac artery and common femoral artery.*

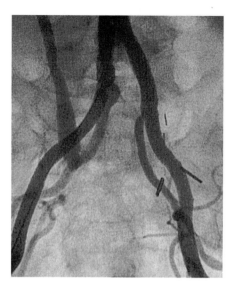

Figure 38.5 *Aortoiliac arteriogram after stenting of both external iliac arteries. The angiogram demonstrates complete elimination of the dissection plane in the right external iliac artery and wide patency bilaterally.*

Final angiography of each limb demonstrated widely patent common and external iliac arteries and normal distal run-off (Figures 38.5). The arterial sheaths were withdrawn immediately and hemostasis was achieved using manual compression. On the next day the patient had normal peripheral pulses and was asymptomatic with ambulation. He was dismissed on aspirin 325 mg/day and clopidogrel 75 mg/day. He remains asymptomatic 3 months later.

Commentary

This case illustrates several interesting features of stenting for iliac arterial occlusive disease. The case description begins with a 'simple' example of focal aortoiliac occlusive bifurcation disease approached with balloon-expandable stents. Although the angiographic result was excellent, the patient had continued severe symptoms. Repeat arteriography demonstrated focal residual disease of the left external iliac artery and an extensive dissection of the right external iliac artery. The dissection was most probably created by either sheath or catheter introduction. Both the dissection and the focal left external iliac stenosis were not recognized at the time of the original intervention. The presence of the long (25 cm) sheaths at the conclusion of the initial procedure 'masked' the residual disease after otherwise successful stenting of the aortoiliac bifurcation. Although, in general, we exchange for shorter sheaths at the conclusion of the interventional procedure, it was not done in this case. The report concludes with a more 'complex', staged, multi-vessel stent procedure using self-expanding Nitinol stents to address these problems.

Stent-supported reconstruction of the aortoiliac bifurcation is a safe and highly effective interventional technique. In the past, surgical revascularization was

156

predominantly used to treat distal aortic and aortoiliac bifurcation disease. Although highly effective, traditional surgery is associated with morbidity and mortality rates of 8% and 3%, respectively. Percutaneous revascularization for aortoiliac occlusive arterial disease with both angioplasty and stenting represents an excellent alternative, achieving clinical results equivalent to surgery with extremely low complication rates. Henry et al[2] achieved a technical success in 309 of 310 (99.7%) patients treated with the Palmaz stent, a major complication rate of 1% and secondary patency rates of 94% at 4 years.

Ostial iliac occlusive disease typically involves the distal aorta and is often calcified. We prefer to approach aortoiliac bifurcation disease with balloon-expandable stents using the 'kissing' stent technique. By extending the stent into the aorta, the bifucation is effectively reconstructed, often with a 'double-barrel' conformation. Scheinert et al[3] have reported a 24-month primary angiographic patency rate of 87% among a group of patients treated with this technique. Nawaz et al[4] reported favorable clinical outcomes in 87% of treated patients at 36 months.

Self-expanding stents implanted in the iliac artery are also associated with high procedural success rates and sustained clinical benefit. Sapoval et al[5] have reported 4-year primary and secondary patency rates of 61% and 86%, respectively, among a group of patients treated with the self-expanding stainless steel Wallstent (Boston Scientific Medi-Tech, Watertown, MA) in the iliac artery. The self-expanding stent size is generally 1 mm larger than the reference vessel to ensure adequate stent apposition. Post-deployment balloon inflation is almost always performed with self-expanding stents. Predictors of improved long-term patency after aortoiliac stenting include: (1) limited femoropopliteal disease, (2) use of aspirin and (3) a post-procedural pressure gradient of less than 10 mmHg.

References

1. Farrell O, Medelsohn MD, Renato M et al, Kissing stents in the aortic bifurcation. *Am Heart J* 1998;**136**:600–5.

2. Henry M, Amor M, Ethevenot G et al, Palmaz stent placement in iliac and femoropopliteal arteries:primary and secondary patency in 310 patients with 2–4 year follow-up. *Radiology* 1995;**197**:167–74.

3. Scheinert D, Schroder M, Balzer JO et al, Stent-supported reconstruction of the aorto-iliac bifurcation with the kissing technique. *Circulation* 1999;**100**(suppl):11295–300.

4. Nawaz S, Cleveland T, Gaines P et al, Aortoiliac stenting, determinants of clinical outcome. *Eur J Vasc Endovasc Surg* 1999;**4**:351–9.

5. Sapoval MR, Chatellier G, Long AL et al, Self-expandable stents for the treatment of iliac artery obstructive lesions: long-term success and prognostic factors. *Am J Roentgenol* 1996;**5**:1173–9.

CASE 39: STENTING OF THE INFRARENAL AORTA

Ramin Alimard, Evelyne Goudreau,
Michael J Cowley

Background

A 53-year-old white woman with a history of tobacco abuse, systemic lupus erythematosus and hypertension presented with severe bilateral claudication involving the buttocks and thighs. A Doppler study of the segmental lower extremity arteries indicated significant aortoiliac obstruction with ankle brachial indices of 0.41 for the right and 0.44 for the left lower extremity.

Procedure

A retrograde femoral approach was used and access to the aorta was achieved successfully using a 0.038-inch guidewire. An abdominal aortogram revealed a very eccentric high-grade obstruction of the distal aorta, after the origin of the inferior mesenteric artery (Figures 39.1 and 39.2). Intravascular ultrasonography (IVUS) was performed using a Sonicath 9-MHz imaging catheter (Boston

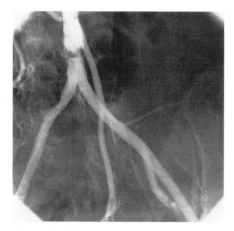

Figure 39.1 *Anteroposterior view of the distal abdominal aorta shows a very-high-grade and eccentric lesion distal to the origin of the inferior mesenteric artery.*

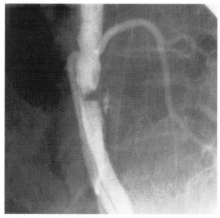

Figure 39.2 *The lateral view of the descending aorta shows the severe eccentric narrowing below the inferior mesenteric artery.*

Scientific Corp., Watertown, MA, USA) and confirmed the severe focal narrowing of the distal aorta. The diameter of the diseased segment by angiography was 9 mm. Both common iliac arteries were free of significant disease.

Angioplasty of the distal aorta was performed using a 12 mm × 20 mm Medi-Tech balloon catheter (Boston Scientific Corp.) inflated to 2 atm. Repeat angiography showed significant improvement of luminal diameter with evidence of a linear dissection and a luminal filling defect (Figure 39.3). A Palmaz P188 stent (Cordis, Miami, FL) was manually mounted on the 12 mm × 20 mm balloon catheter after removal of the hydrophilic coating of the balloon with alcohol. Stent deployment was performed slowly, at low inflation pressure. During deployment, the stent was noted to migrate off the balloon and into the right common iliac artery. The stent could not be repositioned and was then deployed in situ, partially extending into the common iliac artery. A second P188 Palmaz stent was deployed across the primary lesion. The balloon was inflated more rapidly to prevent distal migration. Repeat angiography showed excellent angiographic improvement with essentially no residual narrowing in the distal aorta (Figure 39.4). However, there was evidence of dissection of the common iliac artery without luminal compromise.

Commentary

Several small series have reported the safety and efficacy of percutaneous techniques in the treatment of localized obstruction of the infrarenal abdominal

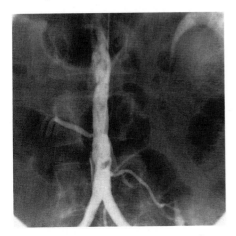

Figure 39.3 *Anteroposterior view after balloon inflation shows improvement in the luminal diameter, but with a filling defect and a linear dissection.*

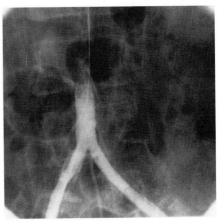

Figure 39.4 *Final angiogram shows excellent result after stenting of the distal aorta. There is evidence of extraluminal dissection of the right common iliac artery without luminal compromise.*

159

aorta in carefully selected patients. Certain technical considerations can be extracted from a review of the published data: the relatively large size of the aorta theoretically increases the risk of rupture with percutaneous interventions at any given pressure because of the increase in wall tension as the diameter increases (law of La Place). Therefore, large vessels can be dilated at lower inflation pressures, but they may also rupture at lower pressures. Pain during balloon inflation should be viewed as an indication of overstretching the arterial wall with risk of rupture. Fortunately, there has been only one case report of rupture of the aorta after balloon angioplasty.

Involvement of the inferior mesenteric artery is not an absolute contraindication to percutaneous treatment. There have been no reports of mesenteric ischemia associated with balloon angioplasty or stenting in the region of the inferior mesenteric artery, although bowel ischemia is a theoretical concern and patency of the superior mesenteric, celiac and hypogastric arteries should be documented.

Calcified or highly eccentric lesions should be approached with caution because they are less likely to respond favorably to balloon angioplasty and have an increased risk of complications. Complex lesions should have better outcomes with stenting. In the case presented here, the eccentricity and calcification may have contributed to the distal migration of the stent. Similarly, one case of stent displacement has been reported secondary to elastic recoil at a proximal aortic anastomosis of a prosthetic graft. The newer self-expanding stents may be a better choice for such lesions, and some of them allow for repositioning when needed, before full deployment.

It is unclear whether all lesions should undergo stent implantation. Stenting is clearly indicated for suboptimal angioplasty results, and seems most appropriate for patients with eccentric or complex lesions. Primary or direct stenting may also be done, and has the theoretical advantage of decreased risk of distal embolization compared with balloon angioplasty. However, embolization is rare with focal obstruction of the distal aorta and this should not be a major consideration.

References

1. Nyman U, Uher P, Lindh M et al, Primary stenting in infrarenal aortic occlusive disease. *Cardiovasc Intervent Radiol* 2000;**23**:97–108.

2. Long AL, Gaux JC, Raynaud AC et al, Infrarenal aortic stents: Initial clinical experience and angiographic follow-up. *Cardiovasc Intervent Radiol* 1993;**16**:203–8.

3. Vorwerk D, Gunther RW, Schurmann K, Wendt G, Aortic and iliac stenoses: Follow-up results of stent placement after insufficient balloon angioplasty in 118 cases. *Radiology* 1996;**198**:45–8.

4. Audet P, Therasse E, Oliva VL et al, Infrarenal aortic stenosis: Long-term clinical and hemodynamic results of percutaneous transluminal angioplasty. *Radiology* 1998;**209**:357–63.

5. Berger T, Sorenson R, Konrad J, Aortic rupture: a complication of angioplasty. *Am J Radiol* 1986;144:1285–6.

6. Westcott MA, Bonn J, Comparison of conventional angioplasty with the Palmaz stent in the treatment of abdominal aortic stenoses from the STAR registry. *JVIR* 1998;**9**:225–31.

Case 40: Gluteal artery stenosis: an unusual cause of claudication

Tyrone J Collins, Rajesh Subramanian,
Christopher J White

Background

A 75-year-old man presented for evaluation of right hip claudication. He had
been having complaints of exertional right hip claudication over the last 2 years
that now occurred when walking less than 100 m. Physical examination and ankle
brachial indices (1.14 bilaterally) were normal. Spinal magnetic resonance
imaging was consistent with spinal stenosis and he underwent surgical repair.
Several months after surgery, he returned with progressive worsening of his right
hip claudication. Aortography with run-off demonstrated several stenoses
involving the branches of the right internal iliac (hypogastric) artery, without
involvement of the aorta, common iliac or external iliac arteries.

Procedure

A 7 Fr sheath was placed in the left common femoral artery and a 4 Fr
multipurpose catheter was advanced into the abdominal aorta. Pressure gradients
were measured between the abdominal aorta and left common femoral artery,
between the left and right common femoral arteries, and between the left
common femoral artery and right internal iliac arteries. This was repeated after
the administration of 30 mg intra-arterial papaverine. No pressure gradients were
found.

High-grade lesions were noted in the branches of the right internal iliac
artery. The right superior gluteal artery was occluded shortly after its origin
from the anterior trunk of the right internal iliac artery; the inferior gluteal
artery and internal pudendal artery also had severe stenoses (Figure 40.1). A 7
Fr Balkan cross-over sheath (Cook, Bloomington, IN, USA) was exchanged for
the 7 Fr sheath in the left common femoral artery. Anticoagulation was obtained
with 5000 IU intra-arterial heparin. A 6 Fr Hockey-Stick coronary angioplasty
guiding catheter was advanced through the crossover sheath to engage the right
internal iliac artery. The right internal pudendal artery stenosis was crossed with

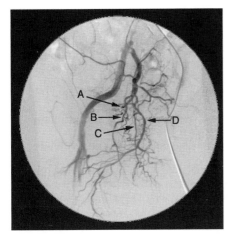

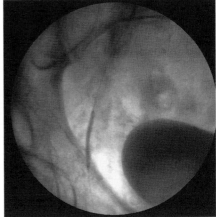

Figure 40.1 *Baseline angiogram demonstrating stenosis involving the branches of the right internal iliac (hypogastric) artery (arrowheads). (a) Right superior gluteal artery; (b) right inferior gluteal artery; (c) right internal pudendal artery; (d) right middle rectal artery.*

Figure 40.2 *Balloon dilatation of the right internal pudendal artery.*

an 0.014-inch Spartacore guidewire (Guidant, Santa Clara, CA) and dilated with a 2.5 mm × 30 mm Crossail balloon (Guidant) (Figure 40.2). As a result of a post-dilatation stenosis of 30% or more, two coronary stents, 3 mm × 23 mm and 2.5 mm × 28 mm Tetra (Guidant), were deployed at 10 atm. Next, the total occlusion of the right superior gluteal artery was crossed with the 0.014-inch Spartacore wire (Figure 40.3). A 3 mm × 13 mm Tetra stent (Figure 40.4) was

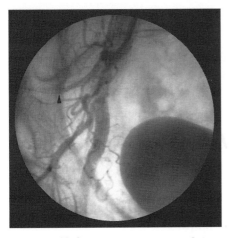

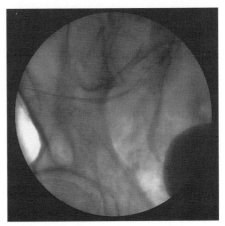

Figure 40.3 *The total occlusion of the right superior gluteal artery crossed with a 0.014-inch Spartacore wire (arrowhead).*

Figure 40.4 *Balloon dilatation of the right superior gluteal artery.*

163

deployed. Finally, after pre-dilatation a 3 mm × 23 mm Tetra stent was placed at the stenosis with excellent result (Figure 40.5). Final angiography demonstrated excellent flows, with resolution of the stenosis in the right internal pudendal artery and in the right superior and inferior gluteal arteries (Figure 40.6). The patient was discharged the next day and the following day, for the first time in years, he walked a mile without symptoms.

Commentary

This case illustrates that not all cases of 'spinal stenosis' can explain a patient's symptoms. The patient underwent surgical correction of his spinal stenosis for 'pseudoclaudication' because there was no objective evidence of lower extremity ischemia. When spinal surgery failed to relieve his progressive and disabling symptoms, he underwent angiography, which finally revealed the 'culprit' lesions in the branches of the internal iliac artery.

Hip claudication is a known manifestation of arterial occlusive disease involving the internal iliac artery. It is important to recognize that debilitating hip or buttock claudication may occur in the presence of normal or only mildly abnormal common femoral pulses and ankle brachial index, as a result of isolated involvement of the internal iliac artery and/or its branches (superior and inferior gluteal arteries). Aortography is the only modality that will make the diagnosis when the terminal aorta, common iliac, external iliac and common femoral arteries are normal or only mildly diseased.

Percutaneous angioplasty and/or stenting from the contralateral femoral access is an effective treatment and should be considered as first-line therapy in the

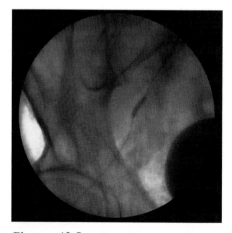

Figure 40.5 *Balloon dilatation of the right inferior gluteal artery.*

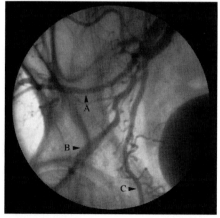

Figure 40.6 *Final angiogram demonstrating excellent flows in (a) the right superior gluteal artery, (b) the inferior gluteal artery and (c) the right internal pudendal artery.*

164

management of this syndrome. In these smaller diameter vessels we prefer to use coronary equipment.

References

1. Iwai T, Sato S, Sakurazawa K et al, Hip pain caused by buttock claudication. Relief of symptoms by transluminal angioplasty. *Clin Orthop* 1992;**284**:176–80.

2. Batt M, Desjarjin T, Rogopolos A et al, Buttock claudication from isolated stenosis of the superior gluteal artery. *J Vasc Surg* 1997;**25**:584–6.

3. Cook AM, Dyet JE, Percutaneous angioplasty of the superior gluteal artery in the treatment of buttock claudication. *Clin Radiol* 1990;**41**:63–5.

CASE 41: FEMORO-POPLITEAL ARTERY ANGIOPLASTY

Christopher J White

Background

A 58-year-old woman was referred from her primary care physician for evaluation of left lower extremity pain with walking. She has no prior history of coronary or vascular disease, and her only risk factor for atherosclerotic disease was a positive family history. She reports progressive worsening of left calf pain after walking less than one block. The pain began 1 month ago and has gradually worsened.

On physical examination her left popliteal, posterior tibial and dorsalis pedis pulses are severely diminished. Her ankle brachial index (ABI) on the left is 0.58 at rest. Doppler ultrasonography reveals a velocity step-up at the popliteal artery consistent with a discrete stenosis. Diagnostic angiography with possible ad hoc intervention is planned.

Procedure

Contralateral access via the right common femoral artery with a 6 Fr sheath is obtained. Abdominal aortography with run-off was performed with a 6 Fr pigtail catheter. Next an internal mammary artery catheter was placed into the left common iliac artery over an 0.035-inch glidewire (Terumo: Boston Scientific Corp., Watertown, MA, USA). An exchange length extra-stiff 0.035-inch Amplatz (Cook, Bloomington, IN) wire was advanced through the internal mammary catheter to the left common femoral artery. A 6 Fr Balkan (Cook) crossover sheath was then advanced over the Amplatz wire to the common femoral artery and 5000 IU heparin were given.

Selective angiography demonstrated a 99% stenosis in the popliteal artery (Figure 41.1) with normal run-off below the knee. The lesion was crossed with

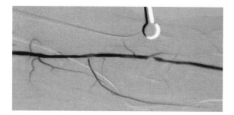

Figure 41.1 Baseline angiogram of the left femoro-popliteal arteries with a tight stenosis. The metallic artefact in the picture is a reference object for quantitative measurements of the vessel diameter.

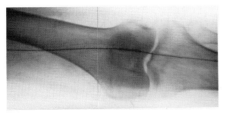

Figure 41.2 *Balloon inflation in the lesion.*

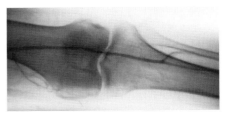

Figure 41.3 *Final angiography.*

an 0.035-inch Wholey (Malinckrodt, St. Louis, MO) wire and dilated with 4 mm × 20 mm Opta-5 (Cordis) balloon at 6 atm (Figure 41.2). The angiographic result after balloon angioplasty was excellent with less than 10% residual stenosis (Figure 41.3).

The catheters and sheaths were removed and the access closed with a 6 Fr Perclose device. The patient was ambulating in 4 hours and discharged home on daily aspirin 325 mg with instructions to return to normal activity. Her post-percutaneous transluminal angioplasty (PTA) ABI on the left was 0.88.

Commentary

Balloon angioplasty has been shown in several randomized trials to achieve equivalent hemodynamic results and long-term patency rates compared with surgery in lesions that are amenable to either therapy. In patients with discrete symptomatic lesions, angioplasty is the preferred therapy over surgery resulting from less morbidity, shorter hospital stay, and equal hemodynamic and durability results. In patients who return with re-stenosis, PTA is usually repeated. although surgery remains an option. One advantage of angioplasty is that it does not 'burn' bridges, allowing for surgery to performed at a later date if required.

Stents have not been shown to improve outcomes after successful angioplasty in the femoro-popliteal vessels. As a result of this, it is our practice to place stents only for failed (residual diameter stenosis ≥ 30% or flow-limiting dissection) angioplasty procedures. This practice has been termed 'provisional stenting'.

CASE 42: ADJUNCTIVE ABCIXIMAB FOR LIMB THREATENING ISCHEMIA

Jose A Silva

Background

A 70-year-old man presents with a 3-day history of left calf pain with coldness and cyanosis of the left foot. He underwent aortobifemoral bypass grafting 5 years ago; 7 months ago he underwent left femoropopliteal bypass grafting with synthetic graft material, which 2 months later required surgical thrombectomy and revision of the distal anastomosis for thrombotic occlusion. Two months before this admission, the femoropopliteal bypass graft had failed again and he underwent a left femoroposterior tibial bypass with a saphenous vein graft.

His vascular surgeon referred him for percutaneous intervention after duplex ultrasonography revealed that the femoroposterior tibial vein graft was occluded. His baseline ankle brachial index (ABI) was 0.2 on the left and normal on the right.

Procedure

Right common femoral artery access was obtained, a 6 Fr Simmons I catheter (Cordis, Miami, FL, USA) was positioned within the left common iliac artery, and a hand injection angiogram identified an occluded graft immediately after the origin of the profunda femoris artery (Figure 42.1).

Using an angled 0.035-inch glidewire (Medi-Tech, Watertown, MA), the occluded graft was successfully entered and the wire was positioned in the distal portion of the graft. The Simmons catheter was then exchanged for a 5 Fr Cobra

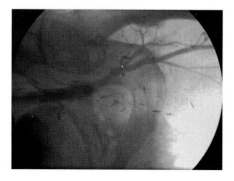

Figure 42.1 Occluded femoroposterior tibial saphenous vein bypass graft at its origin.

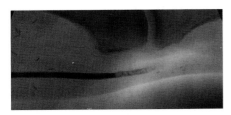

Figure 42.2 *Post-thrombolysis angiogram showing persistent occlusion and a significant thrombus burden in the distal graft.*

catheter which was advanced into the distal portion of the graft. The glidewire was then exchanged for a 0.035-inch extra-stiff Amplatz (Cook, Bloomington, IN) guidewire. A 6 Fr crossover sheath (Cook) was advanced across the aortic bifurcation and positioned proximal to the origin of the graft in the left common femoral artery. A 5 Fr Mewissen perfusion catheter (Medi-Tech) was advanced into the proximal portion of the graft, and a 0.035-inch Katzen wire (Medi-Tech) was positioned through the Mewissen catheter in the distal third of the graft. Heparin 5000 U was administered as a bolus and an infusion at the rate of 500 U heparin/h was started. Urokinase 10 000 U were administered over 10 min (5000 U through the Mewissen catheter and 5000 U through the Katzen wire) directly into the occluded graft. An infusion of urokinase was started at 4000 U/min through the Mewissen catheter and 2000 U/min through the Katzen wire.

After 12 hours angiography revealed resolution of thrombus in the proximal three-quarters of the graft, but there was still a significant amount of thrombus in the distal portion of the graft (Figure 42.2). Mechanical thrombectomy with the Possis AngioJet (Possis Medical, Minneapolis, MN) catheter was performed after the 6 Fr was exchanged for a 8 Fr crossover sheath. The graft was recrossed with a 0.014-inch guidewire and positioned in the posterior tibial artery. Several passes were performed with the AngioJet catheter until no further

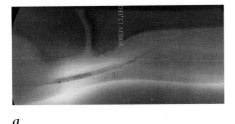

a

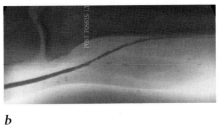

b

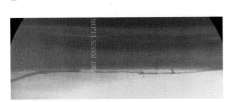

c

Figure 42.3 *(a) Rheolytic thrombectomy of the distal graft, showing the Possis AngioJet catheter. (b) Angiogram after rheolytic thrombectomy, showing almost complete resolution of the thrombus and significant stenosis at the distal anastomosis of the graft with the posterior tibial artery. (c) Severe diffuse disease of the native posterior tibial artery.*

169

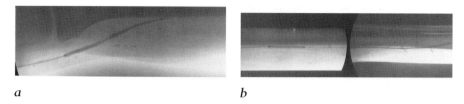

a   *b*

Figure 42.4 *(a) Percutaneous transluminal angioplasty (PTA) of the distal anastomosis of the vein graft and the posterior tibial artery. (b) Top: PTA of the native posterior tibial artery. Bottom: after PTA.*

reduction in the thrombus burden was observed (Figure 42.3).

Figure 42.3 shows almost complete resolution of the thrombus burden, but it should be noted that there is residual stenosis in the distal anastomosis of the graft with the posterior tibial artery, as well as in the native posterior tibial artery. The distal anastomosis was dilated with a 4 mm balloon and the native posterior tibial artery with a 3 mm balloon with an excellent angiographic result (Figures 42.4 and 42.5). There was restoration of the pulse and resolution of the ischemic changes in the left foot. The patient was discharged on aspirin and warfarin (Coumadin).

Approximately 12 hours after discharge, the patient developed recurrent resting limb ischemia and loss of the left posterior tibial pulse. A repeat angiogram confirmed re-thrombosis of the graft (Figure 42.6). Using a Mewissen catheter and a Katzen wire, urokinase was readministered and a bolus (0.25 mg/kg) and 12-hour infusion (0.125 µg/kg per min) of abciximab (Eli Lily, Indianapolis, IN) was begun. Angiography after the 12 hours revealed excellent

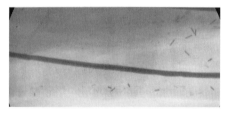

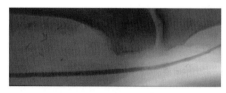

a   *b*

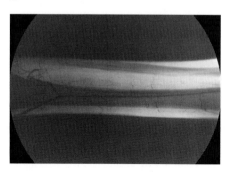

Figure 42.5 *(a) Final angiographic result of the body of the graft. (b) Final angiographic result of the distal anastomosis. (c) Final angiographic result of the native posterior tibial artery.*

c

170

results. The distal anastomosis, as well as the sites that had undergone balloon dilatation in the native posterior tibial artery, remained widely patent and further balloon angioplasty was not performed (Figure 42.7). The patient was discharged the next day on aspirin and warfarin (Coumadin). At the 1-month follow-up, he was asymptomatic with a palpable posterior tibial pulse.

Commentary

Thrombotic lesions present abruptly as a result of either *in situ* thrombosis or arterial embolism from a distant source. *In situ* thrombosis is a far more common cause of acute arterial insufficiency than arterial embolism. It usually occurs in patients with significant atherosclerotic vascular disease or after a plaque ruptures, triggering platelet aggregation and activation of the coagulation system, which ultimately leads to the formation of an obstructive thrombus and acute ischemia.[1]

Embolic occlusion usually originates from a cardiac source, particularly in patients with chronic atrial fibrillation and/or left ventricular thrombus, prosthetic cardiac valves and bacterial endocarditis, among others.[2] In bypass grafts, poor distal run-off is also a frequent cause of graft thrombosis.[3]

This is a case of limb-threatening ischemia caused by thrombotic occlusion of the femoroposterior tibial vein graft as a result of poor run-off. The patient had significant stenosis at the distal anastomosis of the bypass graft, as well as a diffusely diseased native posterior tibial artery. The graft was successfully recanalized with a local infusion of urokinase. To improve the outflow, the anastomosis and the native posterior tibial artery were successfully dilated.

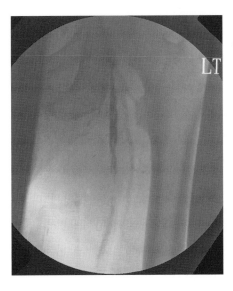

Figure 42.6 *Re-thrombosis of the femoroposterior tibial graft.*

171

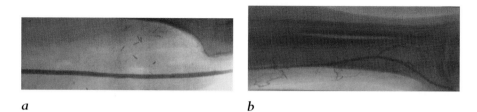

a   *b*

Figure 42.7 (a) Angiography of the femoroposterior tibial graft after successful abciximab and thrombolysis, showing an excellent result. (b) Angiography of the native posterior tibial artery after successful abciximab and thrombolysis.

Thrombolytic therapy has been shown to yield equivalent amputation-free survival rates when compared with surgical therapy.[4,5] Nevertheless, one of the major inconveniences of thrombolytic therapy is that the patient needs to be infused over 6 or more hours, enhancing risk for bleeding complications and its use in patients with recent surgery or recent percutaneous vascular access.

Mechanical thrombectomy with the Possis AngioJet uses the Venturi–Bernoulli vacuum principle, by which high-speed saline jets create a low-pressure region at the tip of the catheter; this then acts to pull the thrombus from the vessel and propel it from the body. In a study from our institution, 21 patients and 22 limbs with contraindications to thrombolysis, and abrupt thrombotic occlusion causing limb-threatening ischemia, were treated with this device. Relief of ischemic symptoms and restoration of pulsatile flow was attained in 20 limbs (91%). The in-hospital and 6-month limb salvage rates (95% and 89%, respectively) and survival rates (86% and 81%) were excellent. This study showed that the device is very useful for this condition, particularly in patients with contraindications for thrombolytic therapy and/or surgery.[6]

The platelet glycoprotein IIb/IIIa receptor inhibitors have been shown conclusively to be of great benefit when used during percutaneous coronary intervention, decreasing the in-hospital and 1-month major cardiovascular events. The use of these agents as adjuvants to percutaneous intervention in the peripheral vascular circulation has not been addressed yet. After the use of abciximab during the second intervention, the graft remained patent at the 1-month follow-up. We can speculate that the trauma inflicted to the endothelium and the atherosclerotic plaque during balloon angioplasty, and/or the proaggregatory effect of the urokinase, may have led to enhanced platelet activation which was inhibited by abciximab.[7]

It is reasonable to suspect that platelets play a crucial role in thrombus formation in the peripheral vascular circulation, and that, similar to the coronary circulation, the use of potent platelet inhibitors such as the group glycoprotein IIb/IIIa glycoprotein inhibitors might decrease the procedural complications.[8]

References

1. Brewster DC, Acute peripheral arterial occlusion. *Cardiol Clin* 1991;**9**:497–513.

2. Abbott WM, Maloney RD, McCabe CC, Lee CE, Wirthlin LS, Arterial embolism: a 44 year perspective. *Am J Surg* 1982;**143**:460–4.

3. Gibson KD, Caps MT, Gillen D et al, Identification of factors predictive of lower extremity vein graft thrombosis. *J Vasc Surg* 2001;**33**:24–31.

4. Ouriel K, Veith FJ, Sasahara AA, for the Thrombolysis or Peripheral Arterial Surgery (TOPAS) Investigators, A comparison of recombinant urokinase with vascular surgery as initial treatment for acute arterial occlusion of the legs. *N Engl J Med* 1998;**338**:1105–11.

5. Ouriel K, Shortell CK, DeWeese JA et al, A comparison of thrombolytic therapy with operative revascularization in the initial treatment of acute peripheral arterial ischemia. *J Vasc Surg* 1994;**19**:1021–30.

6. Silva JA, Ramee SR, Collins TJ et al, Rheolytic thrombectomy in the treatment of acute limb-threatening ischemia: immediate results and six-month follow-up of the multicenter AngioJet registry. *Cathet Cardiovasc Diag* 1998;**45**:386–93.

7. Kawano K, Aoki I, Aoki N et al, Human platelet activation by thrombolytic agents: effects of tissue-type plasminogen activator and urokinase on platelet surface P-selectin expression. *Am Heart J* 1998;**135**:268–71.

8. Topol EJ, Easton JD, Amarenco P et al, Design of the blockade of the glycoprotein IIb/IIIa receptor to avoid vascular occlusion (BRAVO) trial. *Am Heart J* 2000;**139**:927–33.

Case 43: Common femoral artery dissection and repair

Rajesh M Dave, Sumeet Sachdev,
Thomas M Shimshak

Background

A 60-year-old woman presented with a 5-month history of severe right lower
extremity claudication (Rutherford class IC). She had an extensive history of
atherosclerotic heart disease and had undergone uncomplicated multi-vessel
coronary angioplasty and stenting via the right femoral arterial approach 7
months earlier.

Two months later she developed severe exertional right hip and calf
discomfort. Peripheral arteriography from the right common femoral artery
demonstrated a discrete stenosis of the right external iliac artery, and this was
successfully dilated and stented with a Palmaz biliary stent. Unfortunately, her
symptoms did not improve.

An abdominal aortogram 2 months later, from the left femoral approach,
demonstrated a patent right external iliac stent and a lengthy dissection distal to
the stent, from the right external iliac to the right common femoral artery. She
was managed medically and had continued claudication at less than 100 feet. She
presented to us for a second opinion 5 months after the onset of right leg
claudication. Her other medical problems included hypertension, smoking and
type 2 diabetes mellitus. Pertinent physical findings included markedly diminished
right femoral pulse with non-palpable right popliteal and pedal pulses.

Procedure

We performed an abdominal aortogram from the left femoral approach using a 6
Fr sheath and pigtail catheter. The abdominal aorta and both common iliac
arteries were normal. Selective cannulation of the right common iliac artery
using a 6 Fr left internal mammary artery (LIMA) diagnostic catheter from the
contralateral approach was performed. Multiple contrast injections were
performed, taking films in both the anteroposterior (AP) and right anterior
oblique (RAO) views to assess the right external and common femoral arteries.

The RAO view demonstrated a complex linear dissection plane encompassing
the right common femoral and external iliac arteries (Figure 43.1). This

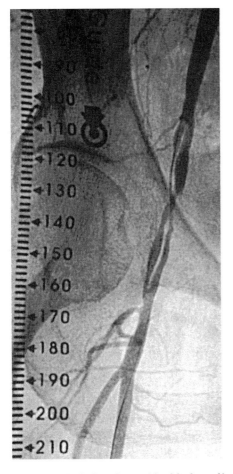

Figure 43.1 Right anterior oblique (RAO) view of right common femoral artery demonstrating a complex 55-cm-long spiral dissection. The true lumen begins at the lateral aspect and 'crosses-over' the dissection plane at the midportion (134 cm mark) and terminates at the distal portion of the common femoral artery (corresponding to the 162 cm mark). There is severe luminal compromise with subtotal obstruction.

dissection had the classic 'double-barrel' appearance, and, frankly, it was difficult to ascertain the true lumen. The distal-most portion of the right common femoral artery (just proximal to the bifurcation of the superficial femoral and profunda femoris artery) was patent without significant disease. The superficial femoral, profunda femoris and distal arterial circulation were well preserved.

We elected to approach the flow-limiting, subtotal, lengthy dissection using a contralateral approach. The patient was given a bolus of 5000 U intravenous heparin. The right common iliac artery was engaged with a 6 Fr Zuma LIMA guide catheter (Medtronic AVE, Minneapolis, MN, USA). We advanced a 0.014-inch Hi Torque Floppy II (Guidant, Advanced Cardiovascular Systems Inc., Temecula, CA) guidewire through the guide, directing the guidewire into what was judged to be the true lumen. At this point, we examined the artery with intravascular ultrasonography (IVUS), tracking a 3 Fr, 40-mHz IVUS catheter over the 0.014-inch guidewire. This provided unequivocal confirmation of the guidewire position within the true lumen and also characterized the extent and relationship of the dissection plane (Figure 43.2).

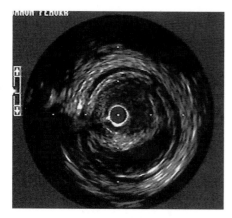

Figure 43.2 Pre-intervention intravascular ultrasound (IVUS) image of the right common femoral artery, demonstrating both true and false luminas, i.e. 'double-barrel' appearance of the dissection.

The vessel was pre-dilated with a 3.5 mm × 40 mm Crosssail (Guidant, Advanced Cardiovascular Systems Inc.) balloon, which was advanced over the 0.014-inch guidewire through the 6 Fr LIMA guide catheter. After pre-dilatation, the 0.014-inch Hi Torque Floppy wire was exchanged for 0.035-inch Wholey Hi-Torque Modified J guidewire (Mallinckrodt Inc., St Louis, MO). The guide catheter was withdrawn over the 0.035-inch wire and the sheath was exchanged for a 6 Fr UP&OVER Balkin contralateral sheath (Cook Inc., Bloomington, IN). An additional series of balloon inflations was then performed using a 4 mm × 10 cm Powerflex plus (Cordis Endovascular, Miami, FL), encompassing the entire

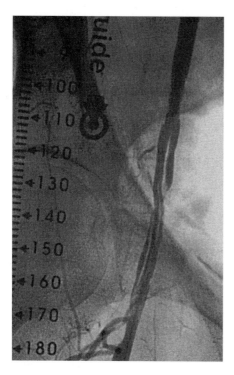

Figure 43.3 Right femoral arteriogram (RAO view) following pre-dilatation with a 4.0 mm balloon catheter. Although the lumen was improved, the results were suboptimal, characterized by a persistent, lengthy dissection plane.

176

length of the dissection plane and the proximal portion of the right external iliac artery stent.

We re-visualized the target segment using AP and oblique views. There was considerable improvement in the appearance of the target region, although the dissection plane had persisted (Figure 43.3). We stented this segment, deploying two sequential 7 mm × 56 mm DYNALINK Biliary Self-expanding stents (Guidant, Advanced Cardiovascular Systems Inc.) over a 0.014-inch Hi-Torque Floppy guidewire. These stents were post-dilated with a 5 mm × 10 cm Powerflex plus balloon (Cordis Endovascular, Warren, NJ) and a 6 mm × 40 mm RX Viatrac 14 balloon (Guidant, Advanced Cardiovascular Systems Inc.).

Repeat angiography was then performed through the contralateral sheath. This demonstrated complete resolution of the dissection plane, wide patency of the external iliac and common femoral arteries, and normal run-off (Figure 43.4).

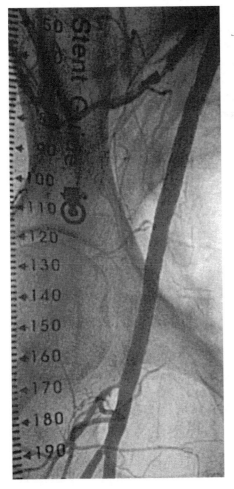

Figure 43.4 Right femoral arteriogram following deployment of two 7 mm × 56 mm DYNALINK Nitinol stents and subsequent angioplasty with 5.0 mm and 6.0 mm balloon catheters.

177

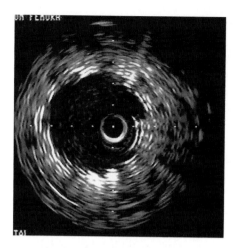

Figure 43.5 Post-stent placement intravascular ultrasound image of right femoral artery.

Repeat ultrasonography examination with the 3 Fr 40-mHz Atlantis IVUS catheter demonstrated obliteration of the dissection plane, complete apposition of the stents and a minimum luminal diameter (MLD) of 4.5–5 mm (Figure 43.5).

Clinically, the right femoral pulse was normal on palpation, having been absent before the expansion of the stents by the interventional procedure. The arterial sheath was withdrawn into the left common femoral artery. After angiographic assessment of the left femoral sheath introduction site, a 6 Fr AngioSeal vascular closure device (St Jude Medical, Diagnostic Division, Minnetonka, MN) was used to achieve hemostasis. The patient was asymptomatic on the following day and was discharged from the hospital on aspririn 325 mg/day and clopidogrel 75 mg/day).

Commentary

This case summarizes the approach to a patient with a complex, flow-limiting, spiral dissection of the right common femoral and external iliac arteries. The dissection was probably precipitated by guidewire, sheath and/or catheter manipulation 5 months earlier. The initial angiogram and percutaneous intervention were performed using a contralateral approach because of the distal location of the dissection. The initial angiogram demonstrated very complex anatomy and it was difficult to differentiate the true from the false lumen. The relationship of small side branches and the appearance of the proximal and distal ends of the spiral dissection provided insight into identifying the true lumen.

As a result of the complexity of the dissection, we initially used a highly steerable and relatively atraumatic 0.014-inch guidewire. Using this guidewire we were able to negotiate the vessel easily, tracking the guidewire into the distal common femoral artery and proximal superficial femoral artery. Final confirmation of the guidewire position was provided by interrogation with IVUS.

Once the anatomy was clarified, the intervention was initiated. We used a low-profile coronary balloon catheter initially, which was intentionally sized conservatively (4.0 mm diameter). This was followed by deployment of Nitinol, self-expanding stents to encompass the entirety of the dissection plane. Post-deployment dilatation with 5 mm and 6 mm balloon catheters was performed, and the final angiogram demonstrated wide patency with complete resolution of the dissection.

The incidence of limb-threatening complications of the arterial access site is infrequent. Bogart et al[1] reported the results of a prospective randomized trial assessing femoral arterial complications after cardiac catheterization among 503 consecutive patients. They identified a 0.4% incidence of limb ischemia and thrombosis of the femoral artery. Clinical assessment, including non-invasive arterial duplex scanning, can assist in the evaluation of a patient with diminished post-procedure femoral pulse(s). Ultimately, arteriography (usually from the contralateral approach) clarifies the diagnosis and defines treatment options.

References

1. Bogart DB, Bogart MA, Miller JT et al, Femoral artery catheterization complications: A study of 503 consecutive patients. *Cathet Cardiovasc Diagn* 1995;**34**:8–13.

2. Oweida SW, Roubin GS, Smith RBD et al, Postcatheterization vascular complications associated with percutaneous transluminal coronary angioplasty. *J Vasc Surg* 1990;**12**:310–15.

3. Waxman R, King SBr, Douglas JS et al, Predictors of groin complications after balloon and new device coronary intervention. *Am J Cardiol* 1995;**75**:886–9.

Case 44: Long superficial femoral artery occlusion and laser-assisted angioplasty

William B Abernathy, Laura Berke,
Kenneth Rosenfield

Background

A 65-year-old man with type 1 diabetes presented with severe cardiomyopathy (ejection fraction of 15%), ulcerative colitis (treated with ileostyomy/colectomy), history of possible upper extremity cholesterol embolization after a thrombus embolectomy, and severe peripheral vascular disease. He had previously undergone percutaneous revascularization and thrombolytic therapy of his left leg, which salvaged a threatened limb. Fifteen months ago, he underwent a left femoral-to-popliteal, reversed saphenous vein bypass graft as a result of recurrent ischemic rest pain and left foot ulcers. He now presents with severe right calf claudication and rest pain.

Magnetic resonance angiography disclosed an occluded right superficial femoral artery (SFA) and popliteal artery with reconstitution at the level of the trifurcation vessels. The possibility of surgical repair on the right was discussed; however, in view of his cardiac status and other co-morbidities, the patient, his vascular surgeon and his cardiologist were not in favor of this approach. His right foot had progressively worsened, developing skin breakdown of his toes and lateral aspect of the foot. He was under consideration for enrolment in an investigational angiogenesis gene transfer protocol, but the decision was made to attempt revascularization of the entire right SFA and popliteal artery as a 'salvage' procedure.

Procedure

The right common femoral artery was accessed in an anterograde fashion. A short 6 Fr sheath was advanced into the ostium of the right SFA. Angiography demonstrated occlusion of the proximal SFA (Figure 44.1). Despite efforts with several different wires, no guidewire would enter more than 20 mm into the mid-SFA. After upsizing to a 7 Fr sheath, an Excimer laser catheter was then used to create a channel through the SFA and popliteal occlusion into the

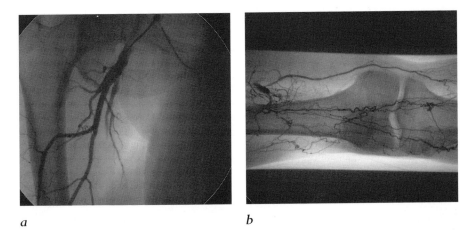

a

b

Figure 44.1 *(a) Angiography via anterograde access of the ipsilateral femoral artery demonstrates occlusion of the superficial femoral artery (SFA). (b) There is only collateral flow to the (c) distal vessels.*

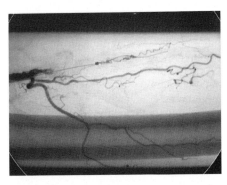

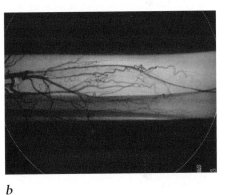

a

b

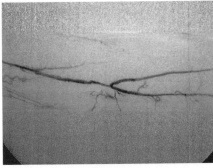

Figure 44.2 *(a) Excimer laser used to develop a channel into the superficial femoral artery (SFA). (b) This device was eventually advanced to the peroneal trunk. (c) Post-laser angiography demonstrates antegrade flow down to the peroneal vessels.*

c

peroneal artery (Figure 44.2). Sequential angioplasties were then performed with a 4 mm × 10 cm balloon at the peroneal trunk and the entire length of the SFA (Figure 44.3). The SFA was further dilated with a 5 mm × 10 cm balloon. An

181

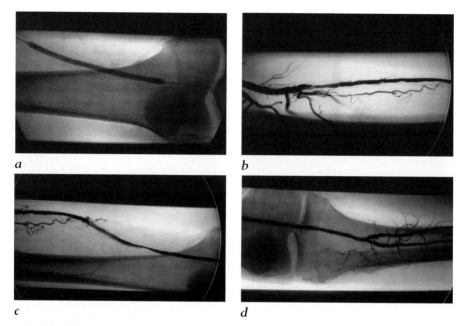

Figure 44.3 (a) Angioplasty of length of superficial femoral artery (SFA) to the peroneal trunk. (b–d) Post-angioplasty films show improvement in the vessel lumen with a dissection in the distal SFA.

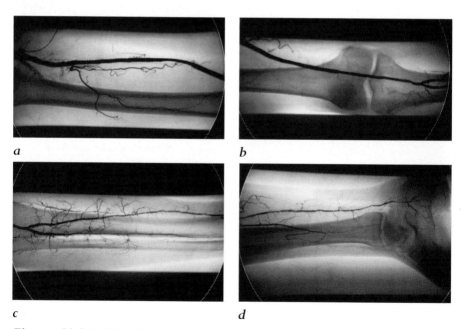

Figure 44.4 (a–d) Final results after implantation of a 6 mm × 12 cm SMART stent in the proximal superficial femoral artery (SFA), and a 7 mm × 11 cm stent in the more distal SFA.

area of dissection in the distal SFA was covered with a 7 mm × 11 cm Memotherm stent, and the more proximal SFA had significant recoil and was covered with a 6 mm × 12 cm SMART stent (Figure 44.4). There was an excellent angiographic result, with less than 20% residual stenosis and good three-vessel run-off.

CASE 45: SUPERFICIAL FEMORAL ARTERY ANGIOPLASTY AND STENTING: A RETROGRADE POPLITEAL APPROACH

Guy N Piegari

Background

The patient is a 69-year-old white man with progressive bilateral two-block claudication. Diagnostic angiography documented a high-grade stenosis of the proximal right common iliac artery and total occlusion of the distal left superficial femoral artery (SFA) with excellent collaterals.

One week after successful right iliac intervention, an attempt to cross the left SFA occlusion anterograde was unsuccessful. Alternative therapies were discussed with the patient and he preferred to proceed with a retrograde popliteal approach.

Procedure

Using a contralateral approach from the right femoral artery, a 6 Fr crossover sheath was placed in the proximal left SFA. The sheath was sutured in place and dressed with a Tegaderm patch. The patient was repositioned in the prone position. Using anterograde injections of contrast via the sheath to locate the popliteal artery, a 5 Fr sheath was placed retrograde into the left popliteal artery (Figure 45.1). The total occlusion was crossed with a 0.035-inch glidewire. The

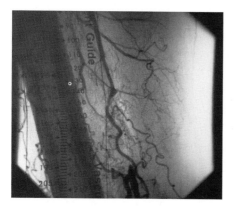

Figure 45.1 *Anterograde contrast injection via the 6 FR sheath placed in the proximal superficial femoral artery and retrograde contract injection from the 5 Fr sheath placed in the popliteal artery demonstrates a 5-cm total occlusion of the distal superficial femoral artery.*

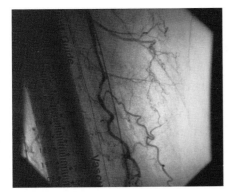

Figure 45.2 *This shows the passage of a wire retrograde from the popliteal artery, which was recognized as being subinimal for a portion of the visualized superficial femoral artery during anterograde contrast angiography. The tip of the wire was thought to be in the true lumen.*

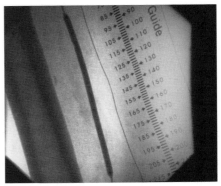

Figure 45.3 *Balloon angioplasty using a 5 cm × 10 cm balloon.*

distal end of the wire appeared to re-enter the true lumen of the mid-SFA (Figure 45.2). The total occlusion was dilated several times with a 4 cm × 10 cm and a 5 cm × 10 cm balloon (Figure 45.3). Anterograde flow was re-established although it was sluggish (Figure 45.4). There was presumed to be long, flow-limiting dissection. The 5 Fr popliteal sheath was exchanged for a 7 Fr sheath and the SFA lesion was stented with a self-expanding Nitinol stent, but there was no anterograde flow. It was now recognized that the glidewire may not have entered the true lumen after crossing the occlusion, and a persistent subintimal was apparent. Vigorous attempts to re-enter the true lumen from the popliteal approach failed. The popliteal sheath was then sewn in place, a Tegaderm dressing was applied and the patient was placed in the supine position.

Selective angiography in an anterograde fashion using a contralateral approach

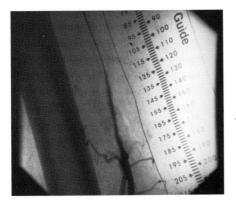

Figure 45.4 *Retrograde contrast angiography demonstrated washout consistent with anterograde flow through the portion of previous total occlusion. However, this flow was quite slow and presumed to be secondary to an intimal flap (long dissection).*

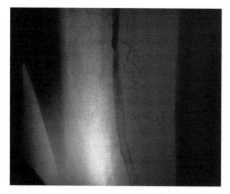

Figure 45.5 *Anterograde contrast angiography documented no flow beyond the stent as the result of an intimal flap.*

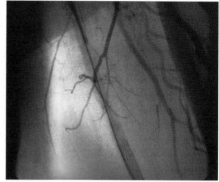

Figure 45.6 *Multiple attempts to cross the intimal flap in an anterograde fashion were unsuccessful. Regardless of the wire used, it preferentially chose the true lumen, which was now obliterated by the stent.*

demonstrated no anterograde flow beyond the proximal portion of the stent (Figure 45.5). Multiple attempts to gain access to the stent lumen were unsuccessful (Figure 45.6). Finally, a 5 cm × 10 cm balloon was advanced anterograde to the stent and inflated to 3 atm (Figure 45.7). With the balloon inflated in the lumen of the SFA, the wire was able to penetrate the flap and enter the stent lumen. With anterograde flow re-established, the balloon was advanced to the proximal portion of the stent and inflated several times up to a maximum of 8 atm. The balloon was then exchanged for an 8 mm × 10 cm self-expanding stent, which was deployed in the proximal SFA overlapping the initial stent (Figure 45.8). Selective angiography of the SFA and distal run-off documented excellent anterograde flow without residual stenosis, dissection or thrombus. The sheath in the right common femoral artery was pulled and the artery was closed with an Angio-Seal device. The popliteal sheath was pulled and hemostasis was obtained with hand pressure.

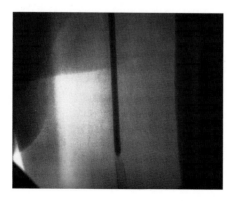

Figure 45.7 *The 5 cm × 10 cm balloon inflated to 3 atm just proximal to the intimal flap.*

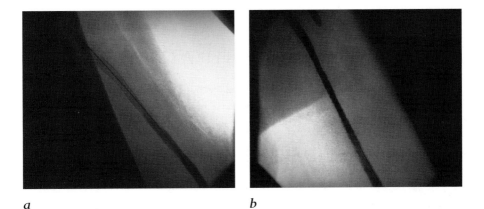

a   *b*

Figure 45.8 *(a) Passage of the wire anterograde through the intimal flap, followed by deployment of a balloon-expandable stent. (b) Re-establishment of anterograde flow via the proximal left superficial femoral artery.*

Commentary

There are three interesting aspects to this case. First, the SFA can be approached using an anterograde or retrograde approach. The retrograde approach may be more challenging for the operator and more difficult for the patient in the prone position, but it will often allow occlusions to be crossed that have failed anterograde attempts.

Second, there is a need to be very cautious about the location of the tip of the wire. Although it is not unusual for a wire to be passed subintimally when crossing occlusions, it is important to confirm that the wire has re-entered the true lumen before performing angioplasty and stenting.

Finally, this case was unique in that a false lumen was stented to the point where there was an intimal flap obstructing anterograde flow. This intimal flap could not be crossed from a retrograde or anterograde approach using the usual techniques. From an anterograde approach, all wires tended to follow the true lumen which was now compressed by the stent (see Figure 45.6). By positioning an inflated balloon just proximal to the intimal flap, the intimal flap could be penetrated with a guidewire, regaining access to the stent lumen.

The patient has been followed for 30 months. He remains free of claudication symptoms and surveillance Doppler studies of the left SFA continue to demonstrate patency with excellent anterograde flow.

Case 46: Below-Knee Intervention for Limb-Theatening Ischemia

John Laird

Background

A patient presented with limb-threatening ischemia of the right lower extremity with a non-healing ulcer on the right foot.

Procedure

Contralateral femoral access of the left common femoral artery was obtained with a 6 Fr sheath. Using a 6 Fr internal mammary artery (IMA) diagnostic catheter and an 0.035-inch Glidewire (Terumo: Boston Scientific Corp. Watertown, MA, USA) the contralateral common iliac artery was cannulated and the glidewire was advanced to the right common femoral artery. Right leg angiography was performed which demonstrated a patent superficial femoral artery (SFA), but with a tight anterior tibial stenosis (Figure 46.1) and an occlusion of the dorsalis pedis artery (Figure 46.2).

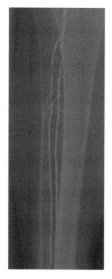

Figure 46.1
Angiography of the left lower leg showing a 90% stenosis of the left anterior tibial artery, a patent peroneal artery and proximal occlusion of the posterior tibial artery.

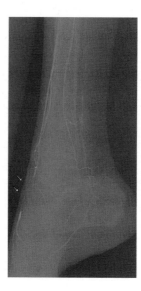

Figure 46.2
Angiography of the left foot showing subtotal occlusion of the dorsalis pedis artery (arrows). Note filling of the distal posterior tibial artery via the collaterals.

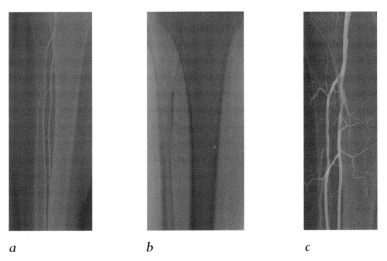

Figure 46.3 *(a) Baseline left anterior tibial stenosis; (b) balloon inflation; (c) final result after balloon dilatation.*

An extra-stiff 0.035-inch Amplatz guidewire (Cook, Bloomington, IN) was advanced through the IMA diagnostic catheter to the proximal left SFA. The IMA catheter and 6 Fr short sheath were exchanged over the extra-stiff Amplatz wire for a 6 Fr Balkan (Cook) crossover sheath. A bolus of 5000 IU heparin was given intra-arterially. A 6 Fr multipurpose coronary guiding wire was then advanced to the popliteal artery through the crossover sheath. The anterior tibial lesion was crossed with an 0.014-inch PT graphics guidewire and dilated with a 3.5 mm × 30 mm Savvy balloon (Figure 46.3).

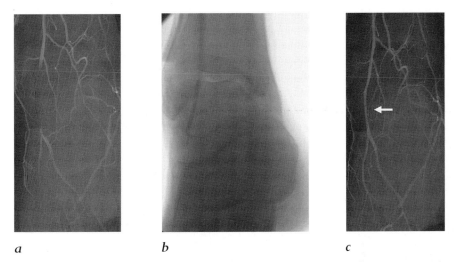

Figure 46.4 *(a) Angiogram of left dorsalis pedis stenosis with wire across lesion; (b) balloon dilatation; (c) post-percutaneous transluminal angiography result.*

189

Next the 0.014-inch PT graphics guidewire was advanced across the dorsalis pedis occlusive lesion. This was dilated with a 2.5 mm × 30 mm long shaft coronary balloon with an excellent result (Figure 46.4). The catheters were removed and the sheath was removed with manual hemostasis.

The patient tolerated the procedure well and was noted to have a palpable dorsalis pedis pulse after the above healing of the right foot ulcer occurred.

Commentary

One of the key principles of below knee intervention for critical limb ischemia is that 'straight line' flow to the foot must be achieved for clinical success and tissue healing to occur. In this case, the dorsalis pedis artery was occluded and treatment of the more proximal anterior tibial artery alone would have likely failed to result in tissue healing. Close attention to the status of the pedal arch is crucial in these cases.

This case also illustrates the contralateral lower extremity use of extra-long coronary equipment to work below the knee. The advantages of this approach include the ability to perform a diagnostic angiogram and to proceed with intervention at the same setting. At the end of the case, hemostasis can be obtained without jeopardizing the treated lesions. The one disadvantage is that extra-long catheters are needed to work below the knee and at the foot.

CASE 47: COMMON FEMORAL ARTERY TOTAL OCCLUSION

Thomas R Gehrig, Harry R Phillips,
James P Zidar

Background

A 46-year-old female nurse with hypertension, a smoking history of 40 pack-years and an extensive family history of peripheral vascular disease presented to her local physician with 8 weeks of right leg claudication and a poorly healing right foot laceration. Poor pedal pulses were noted on physical examination and verified with a resting right ankle brachial index (ABI) of 0.51. Abdominal aortography revealed mild aortic atherosclerotic changes with a total occlusion of the right common femoral artery (CFA), extending to the level of the profunda femoris and superficial femoral artery (SFA) bifurcation (Figure 47.1). Options for revascularization were discussed with the patient who elected for a percutaneous approach.

Procedure

The patient was brought to the peripheral vascular suite 1 week later. Access was obtained with a 6 Fr sheath through the left femoral artery. Heparin was administered to obtain an activated whole blood clotting time (ACT) of 265 s.

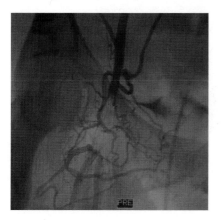

Figure 47.1 *Abdominal aortogram with run-off showing complete occlusion of the right common femoral artery and reconstitution of the right profunda femoris and right superficial femoral artery from ipsilateral collaterals.*

Aortography with run-off showed minimal disease of the popliteal and tibioperoneal vessels of the right leg. The left leg had insignificant disease.

From the left femoral sheath, a 0.035-inch guidewire was advanced through a 5 Fr RDC (Cordis, Miami, FL, USA) angiographic catheter over the aortic bifurcation and into the right external iliac artery. With the wire in place, the RDC catheter and short 6 Fr sheath were removed and a 6 Fr 55-cm Arrow sheath (Arrow, Reading, PA) was advanced over the aortic bifurcation to the level of the right external iliac artery. A 5 Fr multipurpose catheter (Cordis) was advanced to the right external iliac artery and a hydrophilic 0.035-inch Glidewire (Medi-Tech, Waterton, MA) was used to probe the lesion and ultimately advance across the obstruction into the distal SFA. The multipurpose catheter was advanced over the wire into the SFA, and the 0.035-inch Glidewire was removed. A SPARTACORE 0.014-inch wire (Guidant, Temecula, CA) was advanced into the SFA and the multipurpose catheter removed.

With the 0.014-inch guidewire in place, a VIATRAC 6 mm × 40 mm balloon (Guidant) was placed in the obstruction and dilated at 2 and 5 atm (Figure 47.2). Repeat angiography revealed dissection and/or thrombus within the CFA and SFA. A bolus of intravenous abciximab 0.25 mg/kg was administered with additional heparin. A continuous infusion of abciximab was started at 10 μg/min. Repeat angiography continued to demonstrate evidence of lesion disruption (Figure 47.3). A Target sidehole infusion catheter (Medi-Tech, Cork, Ireland) was placed into the lesion and intra-arterial tissue plasminogen activator (tPA) of 20 mg was administered locally over 10 min. Repeat angiography showed little change, and therefore the filling defects were considered to represent local dissection with plaque.

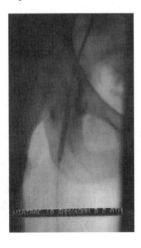

Figure 47.2 *Balloon inflation at the common femoral artery occlusion.*

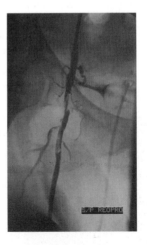

Figure 47.3 *Angiography after balloon dilatation showing disruption of the lesion with filling defects that were thrombi or dissection or both.*

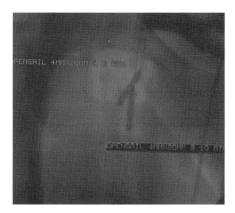

Figure 47.4 Kissing balloons through the DYNALINK stent.

A DYNALINK 6 mm × 33 mm self-expanding Nitinol stent (Guidant) was placed into the common femoral artery, terminating above the origin of the SFA and profunda femoris. An additional 0.014-inch wire was advanced into the profunda. Two OpenSail 4 mm × 20 mm balloons (Guidant) were placed at the SFA/profunda bifurcation in a 'kissing' fashion (Figure 47.4). Repeat angiography showed good flow, but a large plaque burden within the SFA. An additional DYNALINK 5 mm × 28 mm stent was placed into the SFA beyond the profunda ostium. The VIATRAC 6 mm × 40 mm balloon was used to post-dilate both stents.

After removal of the balloon, the patient developed heel pain. Distal injection revealed no evidence of emboli, but repeat iliac angiograms revealed a large thrombus between the stents and dissection distal to the SFA stent, with poor anterograde flow (Figure 47.5). With the patient's pain, poor flow and evidence

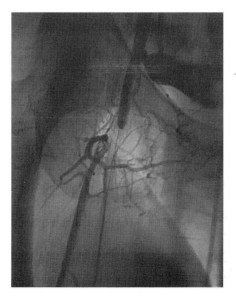

Figure 47.5 Recurrent occlusion distal common femoral artery, between the two stents, with mid-dissection of the superficial femoral artery.

193

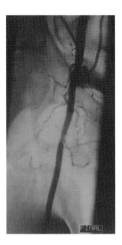

Figure 47.6 *Restoration of straight line flow to the foot with a patent common femoral artery and superficial femoral artery. Note that the profunda femoris artery is now filling from ipsilateral collaterals.*

of dissection, the decision was made to stent across the profunda's ostium. A DYNALINK 6 mm × 28 mm stent was placed in an overlapping fashion between the two previous stents, 'jailing' the profunda. A DYNALINK 6 mm × 56 mm stent was placed distally into the proximal SFA to cover the dissection. Post-dilatation was accomplished with a POWERFLEX 5 mm × 40 mm balloon (Cordis) throughout the stented segment. Final angiography (Figure 47.6) showed excellent flow through the SFA. The profunda had minimal anterograde flow through the jailed ostium, but retained its bridging collaterals. A final distal leg series revealed brisk three-vessel run-off with a possible small embolus in the distal posterior tibial artery. The patient was free of pain at the conclusion of the procedure. The left sheath was removed and the arteriotomy closed with a 6 Fr Perclose device (Perclose, Redwood City, CA). Clopidogrel 300 mg was administered.

The patient was admitted overnight for observation and remained on abciximab and heparin for 12 hours. She was able to ambulate freely without pain on the following morning. Pulses were normal in both lower extremities. She was discharged on clopidogrel 75 mg/day for 1 month, aspirin 325 mg/day indefinitely and an aggressive lipid-lowering regimen. At the two month follow-up, the patient was walking in an unrestricted manner. Pulses remained normal and the resting right ABI was 0.81.

Commentary

This case demonstrates the challenging nature of percutaneous revascularization of common femoral occlusions. Focal common femoral artery occlusion is uncommon in clinical practice. Although acute occlusion may lead to severe ischemic injury, patients usually present with progressive claudication related to inadequate collateralization from the circumflex iliac, circumflex femoral, profunda femoris and hypogastric (internal iliac) gluteal branches. Intervention is indicated for limb-threatening ischemia, resting claudication and, to a lesser extent, exertional claudication refractory to medical therapy. Surgical options include endarterectomy, aortofemoral bypass, axillofemoral bypass, iliofemoral and femorofemoral bypass procedures. Unfortunately, surgery may often be accompanied by significant morbidity in a population that suffers from concomitant coronary and cerebrovascular disease.

In general, percutaneous management of occlusive iliofemoral disease presents concerns over the inability to cross lesions, distal embolization and insufficient compliance of occluded segments to perform angioplasty. Hydrophilic soft-tipped guidewires are often required to cross occlusions. Special care must be taken to avoid subintimal passage and subsequent vessel perforation or rupture. In a study by Vorwerk and colleagues involving 127 patients with iliac occlusions of more than 3 months' duration, mechanical passage through the occlusion was successful in 81% with no incidents of arterial perforation. Peripheral embolic events with percutaneous transluminal angioplasty (PTA) have been reported in 3–17% with surgical intervention required in 1–3%. Some centers recommend the use of periprocedural fibrinolytic therapy, although published rates of embolization are similar, with increases in expense, procedure length and possible bleeding complications. Recently, primary stenting has been advocated to reduce emboli by trapping material against the arterial wall. Regrettably, no direct comparison of primary stenting, adjunctive fibrinolytic therapy, or conventional angioplasty and stenting has been performed. Improved balloon systems and stenting have ameliorated early concerns over non-compliant vessels. Once traversed by a wire, procedural success can be expected in most cases.

Obstruction of the common femoral artery requires special consideration of the initial approach, choice of stent and distal bifurcation issues. Ipsilateral access is generally not possible as a result of the proximity of the lesion. Although an axillary approach has been used, a contralateral femoral access using a long sheath over the aortic bifurcation provides excellent angiographic visualization with ample support and the flexibility to use 8 Fr-compatible devices if necessary. Stent selection must reflect both the anatomic position of the femoral artery, which is subject to forces of both flexion and compression, and the abrupt luminal diameter change that occurs at the femoral bifurcation. Therefore, self-expanding stainless steel or Nitinol stents are preferred, although they possess less radial strength than balloon-expandable stents.

Last of all bifurcation issues provide additional challenges. The profunda femoris serves as the primary blood supply to the thigh, as well as a source of vital collaterals at the level of the popliteal artery during SFA occlusion. Isolated profunda occlusion may cause thigh claudication, but rarely leads to tissue necrosis as a result of the formation of collaterals from the internal iliac and distal circumflex branches. Although not ideal, preservation of the CFA–SFA may require 'jailing' the profunda and reliance on collateral development.

195

References

1. McGovern PJ, Stark KR, Kaufman JL, Rosenberg N, Management of common femoral artery occlusion. *J Cardiovasc Surg* 1987;**28**:38–41.

2. Rutherford RB, Options in the surgical management of aorto-iliac occlusive disease: a changing perspective. *Cardiovasc Surg* 1999;**7**:5–12.

3. Ring E, Freiman D, McLean G, Schwarz W, Percutaneous recanalization of iliac artery occlusions: an unacceptable complication rate. *AJR* 1982;**39**:587–9.

4. Vorwerk D, Guenther R, Schurmann K, Wendt G, Peters I, Primary stent placement for chronic iliac artery occlusions: Follow-up results in 103 patients. *Radiology* 1995;**194**:745–9.

5. Strecker EP, Boos IBL, Hagen B, Flexible tantalum stents for the treatment of iliac artery lesions: long-term patency, complications, and risk factors. *Radiology* 1996;**199**:641–7.

6. Villavicencia R, Meier B, Left axillary approach for balloon recanalization of an occlusion of the right common femoral artery. *Vasa* 1991;**20**:186–7.

Case 48: Femoropopliteal occlusive disease

Jane M Lingelbach, Frank J Criado

Background

A 78-year-old man with hypertension, coronary artery disease, asymptomatic carotid stenosis and tobacco use presented with short-distance claudication of the left calf. Femoral pulses were normal; all distal pulses were absent. There were no lesions on the feet. Doppler examination revealed a resting ankle brachial index (ABI) of 0.64 on the left and 0.90 on the right.

Procedure

Diagnostic angiography revealed a patent aortoiliac system, with a focal stenosis in the right external iliac artery (Figure 48.1a). The right superficial femoral artery (SFA), profunda femoris and popliteal arteries were patent, and there was two-vessel infrapopliteal run-off. The left SFA was calcified with three foci of disease: discrete focal eccentric stenoses proximally and distally, and a segment of disease several centimeters long in the mid-SFA (Figure 48.1b–d). The profunda femoris and popliteal arteries were patent and there was two-vessel infrapopliteal run-off.

Right common femoral artery (CFA) access was obtained and a long 7 Fr sheath was advanced over a guidewire to the right external iliac artery (EIA). Contralateral access to the left common iliac artery (CIA) was achieved with a 5 Fr crossover (CO) catheter and a 0.035-inch Glidewire (Boston Scientific Corp., Watertown, MA, USA), which were advanced to the the distal left EIA. A stiff (Storq: Cordis, Miami, FL) guidewire was then exchanged through the catheter to guide and support advancement of the 7 Fr sheath across the bifurcation and into the left EIA.

Limited subtraction angiography of the femoral bifurcation was obtained to guide selective catheterization of the left SFA, using a 0.018-inch (SV5) guidewire. A 5 Fr flush straight catheter was then advanced over this wire into the proximal SFA and used to obtain a detailed angiographic mask of the vessel (Figure 48.1c). The same 0.018-inch guidewire could be easily advanced across the SFA lesions down to the popliteal artery below the knee. The three areas of stenosis in the proximal, mid- and distal SFA were pre-dilated with a 4-mm small-vessel (Savvy) balloon catheter (Figure 48.2a) and then stented with self-

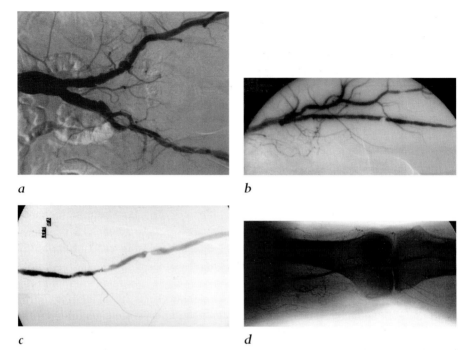

a

b

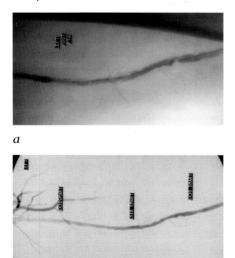

c   d

Figure 48.1 (a) Diagnostic angiography demonstrates a patent aortoiliac system with a focal stenosis in the right external iliac artery. The left SFA is calcified and diffusely diseased, with three foci of disease: (b) discrete focal eccentric stenoses proximally and (c) distally, and a segment of disease several centimeters long in the mid-SFA. (b,d) The profunda femoris and popliteal arteries are patent, and there is two-vessel infrapopliteal run-off. (c) Angiogram obtained via SFA catheterization, for mapping at the time of subsequent intervention.

a

b

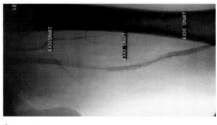

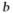

Figure 48.2 (a) After balloon dilatation, the angiographic result is suboptimal. (b) Three discontinuous Nitinol SMART stents were deployed across the three tandem lesions, (c) with a satisfactory angiographic result.

c

198

expanding SMART Nitinol stents. Three separate, non-overlapping, 6-mm-diameter stents were deployed and subsequently post-dilated with a 6-mm balloon catheter. Completion angiography revealed a satisfactory result with rapid flow throughout the SFA/popliteal arteries, with no evidence of dissection and an intact below-knee run-off (Figure 48.2b, c). The sheath was removed over a 0.035-inch Storq guidewire, and the right EIA stenosis was treated with percutaneous transluminal angioplasty (PTA)/stenting on the way out. Hemostasis was achieved with suture-based percutaneous closure using a Perclose device.

After the intervention, the patient was able to ambulate free of claudication, and left pedal pulses were palpable. The left ABI was documented to have increased to 0.80 on the day after the procedure, and was stable 3 months later, at which time duplex imaging revealed turbulent flow and mildly elevated velocities just beyond the proximal SFA stent. Four months after the initial intervention, he returned with clinical evidence of left leg ischemia, and thrombosis of the left SFA was confirmed by non-invasive testing.

Access was obtained via percutaneous retrograde puncture of the right CFA with placement of a 5 Fr introducer sheath over a guidewire. The left CIA was catheterized using a 5 Fr crossover catheter, which was advanced to the level of the left CFA over a 0.035-inch Glidewire (Boston Scientific Medi-Tech). Angiography revealed occlusion of the proximal left SFA extending down to the level of the second stent (in the mid-SFA) (Figure 48.3), with distal reconstitution of the SFA and popliteal artery and maintenance of infrapopliteal run-off. The SFA was re-canalized with a 0.035-inch Storq guidewire, over which a 100-cm-long 5 Fr Mewissen infusion catheter was advanced to reach the distal extent of the thrombosed segment. Through this catheter, intra-arterial infusion of Retavase at 0.5 U/h (in combination with a peripheral intravenous infusion of heparin at 400 U/h) was given. Repeat angiography approximately 16 h later revealed considerable residual thrombus in the proximal/mid-SFA, prompting more proximal repositioning of the infusion catheter. Repeat angiography 8 hours later documented reconstitution of flow through the SFA, but with multiple residual intraluminal defects in the proximal SFA and flow-

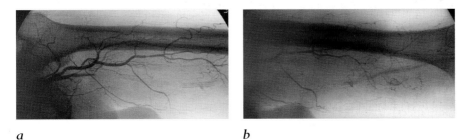

a *b*

Figure 48.3 *At the time of planned intervention, the angiogram obtained via left common femoral injection reveals occlusion of the SFA to the level of the second stent.*

199

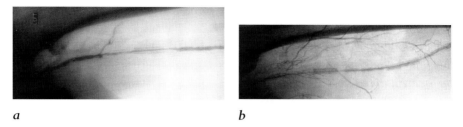

a   *b*

Figure 48.4 *(a) Thrombolysis successfully reconstituted flow through the SFA, with multiple segments of flow-limiting disease and residual intraluminal defects. (b) Angiographic result after suboptimal balloon dilatation.*

limiting disease in the non-stented segments (Figure 48.4a). The thrombolysis catheter was removed, and a long 7 Fr sheath was advanced to the distal left EIA over a 0.035-inch guidewire. A 0.018-inch wire was then advanced across the length of the SFA into the popliteal artery. Balloon dilatation of all segments of residual disease in the SFA was performed with a 5-mm small-vessel balloon (Figure 48.4b), and four additional SMART stents were deployed and post-dilated. On completion, the entire SFA was stented with seven overlapping Nitinol devices (Figure 48.5a). Completion angiography revealed rapid flow throughout the SFA, with a normal appearing lumen (Figure 48.5b), and a patent popliteal artery with unchanged infrapopliteal run-off. The wire, catheter and sheath were withdrawn from the right femoral artery. Puncture-site sealing with a Perclose device completed the procedure.

Left pedal pulses were palpable when the patient was transferred out of the interventional suite. He was maintained on clopidogrel 75 mg/day. Follow-up

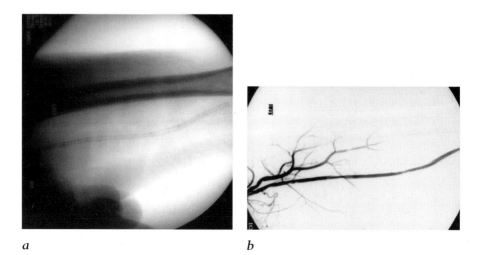

a   *b*

Figure 48.5 *(a) Four additional Nitinol stents were deployed in the SFA, resulting in a total of seven overlapping stents. (b) Completion angiogram reveals a normal flow lumen.*

assessment 1 month later documented that the patient was free of claudication, and the resting left ABI was 0.99.

Commentary

Management of femoropopliteal occlusive disease ranks among the most controversial and least clear areas in the whole of angiology. This case raises a number of interesting issues related to the management of femoropopliteal arterial occlusive disease. What are the appropriate indications for intervention? What are the management options available? If we opt for endovascular intervention, how do we choose the angiographically visualized lesions that need correction versus those that should be left untreated?

What are the appropriate indications for intervention?

Many patients presenting for care have single-level (femoropopliteal) disease and only claudication – not critical ischemia. Although the disease may well show its progressive nature over time, the risk of amputation (or progression to critical ischemia) is low. An exception may be patients with a very low ABI (< 0.5) on presentation; many of these will have multilevel disease. Cessation of smoking and exercise are the mainstays of management. Invasive treatment, either endovascular or surgical, can be justified only in the face of no response to conservative management, significant progression of symptoms or incapacitating claudication with a low ABI. New pharmacological agents have added a new dimension to the power and wisdom of non-interventional management of claudication.

How should we choose between surgical bypass or endovascular intervention?

Results of PTA in the SFA/popliteal territory are well known: mid-term patency rates have been reported to be from mildly acceptable (approximately 50%) to dismal ($< 20\%$). Adjunctive use of first-generation stents (Palmaz and Wallstent) added little if anything to PTA capabilities, with the incremental disadvantage of making potential re-stenoses much more extensive than seen after PTA alone. The concept that stenting in the SFA should be reserved for suboptimal PTA and rescue is a reasonable strategy.

Surgical bypass must still be considered the gold standard in treatment of femoropopliteal occlusive disease. However, 'bypasses' are not all alike, e.g. femoropopliteal bypasses using good-quality saphenous vein graft have proved to be far superior to bypasses made from synthetic grafts. Nevertheless, most surgeons use the synthetic conduit as the initial surgical management of SFA disease in most cases. So the most appropriate surgical yardstick for comparison

201

is the above-knee synthetic femoropopliteal bypass graft, reported to have a long-term patency rate of approximately 50% at 3–5 years, although it is capable of treating short- and long-segment occlusions equally well.

As a generalization, it would seem most appropriate to consider patients for percutaneous endovascular treatment when lesions are focal and less than 7–10 cm in length. More extensive disease should probably be treated by surgical bypass grafting, provided that symptomatology is significant enough to warrant intervention. As an exception to these principles, proponents of the technique of subintimal angioplasty would maintain that even extensive multiple stenoses and occlusions can be treated interventionally, with long-term results that are very similar to surgical outcomes. However, this view and experience are limited to a handful of groups around the world.

Are Nitinol stents better than first-generation devices?

When performing endovascular treatment of SFA disease, how can we decide what lesions to treat versus those that can be left untreated?

Rapidly growing anecdotal reports would seem to support the notion that currently available Nitinol devices fare much better than the Palmaz stent and Wallstent in the SFA. We too have recently become more aggressive with interventional treatment of femoropopliteal disease, it must be understood that this approach is not yet supported by scientifically valid evidence.

This is a significant interventional dilemma, for which there is no clear answer. In spite of significant advances with imaging techniques, including intravascular ultrasonography, we and most other interventionists continue to rely on angiographic appearance for decision-making. As demonstrated in the case reported here, there are times when the whole (or most) of the SFA may need to be treated in order to prevent early failure as a result of the flow-limiting disease that is left behind.

Would it have been better and more cost-effective to treat this patient initially with an above-knee femoropopliteal bypass?

Absolutely!

References

1. Cox GS, Hertzer NR, Young JR et al, Nonoperative treatment of superficial femoral artery disease: Long term follow-up. *J Vasc Surg* 1993;**17**:172–82.

2. Taylor LM, Moneta GL, Porter JM, Natural history and nonoperative treatment of chronic lower extremity ischemia. In: Rutherford RB, ed., *Vascular Surgery*, 5th edn. Philadelphia: WB Saunders, 2000:928–43.

3. Jensen LP, Intermittent claudication. Conservative treatment, endovascular repair or open surgery for femoropopliteal disease. *Ann Chir Gynaecol* 1998;**87**:137–40.

4. Hunink MGM, Donaldson MC, Meyerovitz MF et al, Risks and benefits of femoropopliteal percutaneous balloon angioplasty. *J Vasc Surg* 1993;**17**:183–94.

5. Stanley B, Teague B, Raptis S, Taylor DJ, Berce M, Efficacy of balloon angioplasty of the superficial femoral artery and popliteal artery in the relief of leg ischemia. *J Vasc Surg* 1996;**23**:679–85.

6. Whyman MR, Fowkes FGR, Kerracher EMG et al, Is intermittent claudication improved by percutaneous transluminal angioplasty? A randomized controlled trial. *J Vasc Surg* 1997;**26**:551–7.

7. Vroegindeweij D, Vos LD, Tielbeek AV, Buth J, vd Bosch HC, Balloon angioplasty combined with primary stenting versus balloon angioplasty alone in femoropopliteal obstructions: a comparative randomized study. *Cardiovasc Intervent Radiol* 1997;**20**:420–5.

8. Gray BH, Sullivan TM, Childs MB, Young JR, Olin JW, High incidence of re-stenosis/reocclusion of stents in the percutaneous treatment of long-segment superficial femoral artery disease after suboptimal angioplasty. *J Vasc Surg* 1997;**25**:74–83.

9. Whittemore AD, Belkin M, Infrainguinal bypass. In: Rutherford RB, ed. *Vascular Surgery*, 5th edn. Philadelphia: WB Saunders, 2000: 998–1018.

10. Henry M, Amor M, Beyar R et al, Clinical experience with a new nitinol self-expanding stent in peripheral arteries. *J Endovasc Surg* 1996;**3**:369-79.

Case 49: Excimer Laser-Assisted Recanalization of a Long Superficial Femoral Artery Occlusion

Giancarlo Biamino

Background

A 63-year-old man with known peripheral arterial obstructive disease (PAOD) for 3 years was referred for uncontrolled hypertension and increasing creatinine values. The relative walking capacity was 165 m and the absolute capacity 220 m. The ankle brachial index (ABI) was: at rest, right 0.6, left 0.6; after incomplete treadmill, right 0.4; left 0.4. Magnetic resonance angiography revealed a 90% stenosis of the left renal artery and long occlusions of both superficial femoral arteries (SFAs). In a first step the left renal artery was successfully dilated (Figures 49.1 and 49.2). In the following weeks his blood pressure normalized under medical treatment, with reduced antihypertensive drugs (only an angiotensin-converting enzyme [ACE] inhibitor).

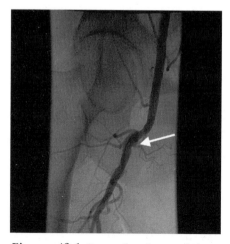

Figure 49.1 *Proximal occlusion of the right superficial femoral artery (SFA). Note the arrow pointing at the 10-mm funnel at the origin of the SFA.*

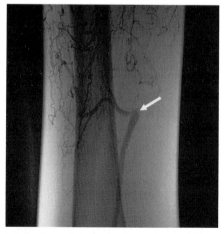

Figure 49.2 *Filling of the distal superficial femoral artery through collaterals. Note the arrow pointing at the distal stump of the occlusion.*

Procedure

First there was placement of an 8 Fr crossover sheath (Cook Inc., Bloomington, IN, USA) from the left common femoral artery into the right external iliac artery. Angiography showed a 10-mm-long funnel after branching of the profunda artery (Figure 49.1). The length of the SFA occlusion was 26 cm (Figure 49.2). The popliteal artery was patent as well as all arteries below the knee (Figure 49.3). Heparin, 5000 IU was administered and an 0.035-inch Terumo (Boston Scientific, Watertown, MA) stiff glidewire was introduced and positioned in the funnel of the right SFA. Using a 2.5-mm Excimer-laser catheter (Spectranetics, Colorado Springs, CO) the 'step-by-step' technique was used to apply laser energy to the occlusion (Figure 49.4).

'Step by step' describes the use of the laser, followed by the advancement of the wire for a few millimeters into the laser channel and again use of the laser until the entire occlusion has been crossed. After the first passage, the 0.035-inch Terumo wire was exchanged for a 0.018-inch wire. The lesion was subjected to the laser for a second time, with continuous flushing of saline through a Y-connector. Subsequently a 5.0 mm × 80 mm balloon was used to dilate the laser channel with pressures up to 12 atm (inflation time 120 s each). Except for a minor dissection in the proximal part of the SFA the angiographic result was excellent (Figures 49.5–49.8). The 8 Fr Perclose device was used to close the puncture site. The patient went home 8 hours later on aspirin 100 mg/day, clopidogrel 75 mg/day for 1 month and low-molecular-weight heparin for 1 month.

At 1 month, duplex ultrasonography confirmed the patency of the right SFA without early re-stenosis. The left SFA was recanalized using the same technique as a few weeks later.

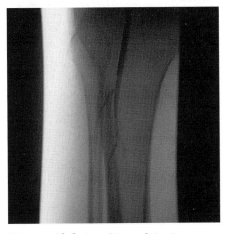

Figure 49.3 *Poor filling of the three patent vessels below the knee before intervention.*

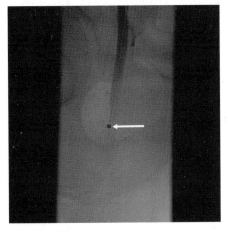

Figure 49.4 *'Step-by-step' technique: note the arrow pointing at the tip of the laser.*

205

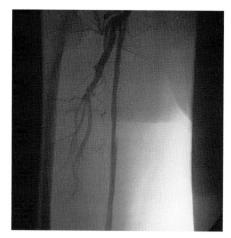

Figure 49.5 *Final result in the proximal superficial femoral artery after treatment with the laser and dilatation using a 5.0 mm × 80 mm balloon.*

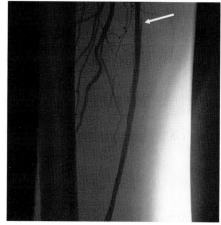

Figure 49.6 *Final result in the medial superficial femoral artery. Note the arrow pointing at the non-flow limiting dissection.*

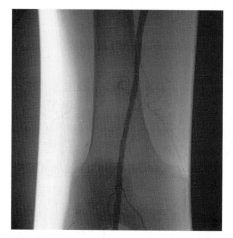

Figure 49.7 *Final result in the distal superficial femoral artery.*

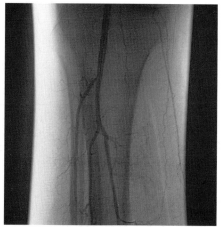

Figure 49.8 *Prompt filling of the vessels below the knee after recanalization of the superficial femoral artery occlusion.*

Commentary

In our experience the use of the 'step-by-step' technique makes laser recanalization of long occlusions both feasible and safe. In addition the secondary patency rate for long femoral occlusions is approximately 75%. It is of the utmost importance to treat the patients with an adequate post-interventional antiplatelet regimen. Furthermore, strict and aggressive follow-up examinations have to be done to detect early re-stenosis.

CASE 50: BELOW-KNEE ANGIOPLASTY

Peter R Vale, Jeffrey M Isner

Background

A 68-year-old white man with coronary artery disease (CAD) who has diabetes and hypertension (treated with coronary artery bypass grafting), smokes and has progressive left calf claudication, presents with rest pain and necrotic ulceration of the left great toe (Figure 50.1). Left popliteal and ankle pulses were not palpable but monophasic by Doppler ultrasound. The ankle brachial index (ABI) on the left was 0.48.

Procedure

Diagnostic lower extremity angiography revealed a high-grade lesion (>80%) of the left superficial femoral artery (SFA) at the level of the adductor canal. The popliteal artery was patent. The tibioperoneal trunk (TPT) was subtotally occluded proximally and severely diseased distally (Figure 50.2). The posterior

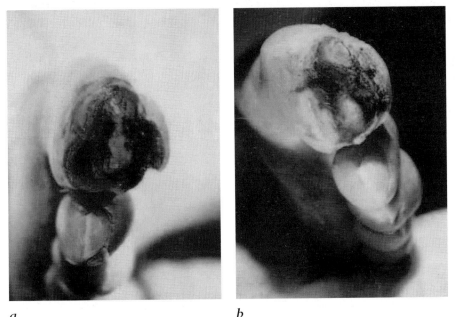

a   *b*

Figure 50.1 *(a–b)Necrotic ulceration of the left great toe.*

tibial (PT) artery was diffusely diseased 2 cm after its origin. The peroneal artery was subtotally occluded at its origin but was reconstituted distally by collaterals and patent to the ankle. The anterior tibial (AT) artery was occluded 2 cm from its origin with no distal filling.

The left common femoral artery was cannulated in an anterograde fashion and a 0.018-inch wire was advanced to the distal popliteal artery. Excimer laser angioplasty achieved minimal improvement in luminal diameter. Next, directional atherectomy was performed and restored near-normal patency. The 0.018-inch wire was then advanced with difficulty through the TPT and into the PT. Excimer laser angioplasty was performed with several passes through the TPT and the proximal PT after which the TPT was widely patent. The wire was then redirected into the peroneal artery and excimer laser angioplasty was again performed in the proximal peroneal artery. Final angiographic images disclosed an excellent result with brisk anterograde flow through the distal popliteal artery, TPT, peroneal and PT arteries (Figure 50.3). The patient's left leg resting ABI increased to 0.87.

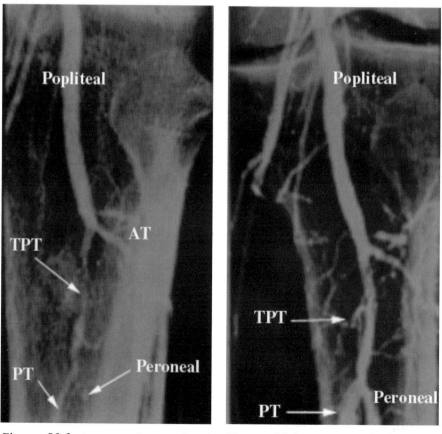

Figure 50.2 *Angiogram showing subtotal occlusion of the tibioperoneal trunk.*

Figure 50.3 *Angiogram after excimer laser angioplasty.*

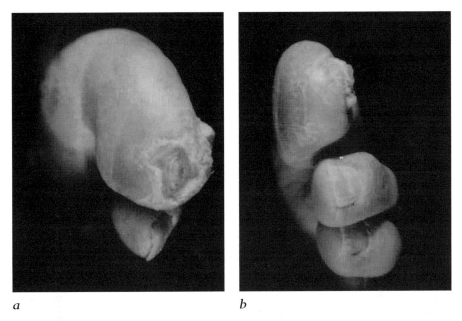

a   *b*

Figure 50.4 *(a–b) Three months after the procedure, showing significant healing.*

Three months after revascularization, there was significant healing of the necrotic ulcer, with only a residual scar (Figure 50.4). However, there had been a deterioration in the resting ABI to 0.57 at the 6-month follow-up,

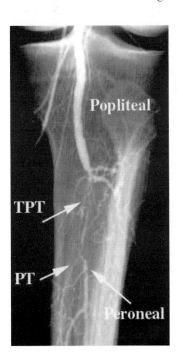

Figure 50.5 *Angiogram at 6 months of follow-up with recurrent tibioperoneal trunk stenosis.*

209

accompanied by recurrent calf claudication. Repeat diagnostic angiography revealed re-stenosis (70%) in the SFA with recurrent infrapopliteal disease. Specifically there was a high-grade stenosis (>90%) of the distal popliteal that also involved a 90% lesion at the origin of the AT (Figure 50.5). The TPT was occluded for 3–4 cm. The peroneal artery was subtotally occluded at its origin but was reconstituted 1 cm further distally by descending geniculate collateral vessels. The PT was subtotally occluded at its origin and diseased throughout with poor distal filling. The AT was occluded 2 cm from its origin with no distal filling.

The left common femoral artery was again entered in an anterograde fashion. A 0.018-inch wire was advanced to the distal popliteal artery. Directional atherectomy was performed on the restenostic SFA lesion achieving excellent luminal patency. A 4 Fr straight catheter was then advanced to the popliteal artery and the 0.018-inch wire was replaced by a 0.009-inch Rotoblator wire, which was advanced with difficulty through the TPT and into the peroneal artery. A 1.5-mm Rotoblator probe was activated and advanced through the TPT

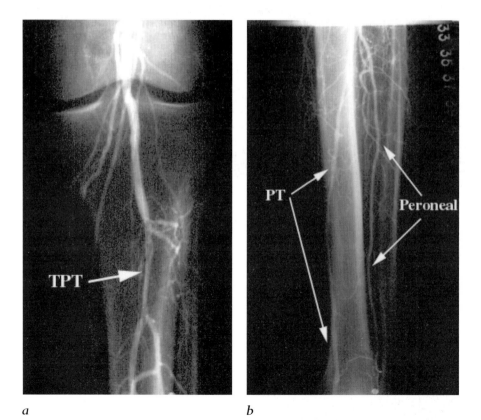

a   *b*

Figure 50.6 (a) Angiogram of the lesion after Rotablator and percutaneous transluminal angioplasty. (b) Angiogram of the distal run-off vessels.

210

and proximal peroneal artery. Angiographic images demonstrated a patent TPT but there was residual haziness present at the lesion. As a result, PTA was performed on the TPT and proximal peroneal artery using a 3 mm × 4 cm balloon. A 0.018-inch wire was directed into the PT and advanced to the ankle joint, after which PTA using a 3 mm × 4 cm balloon was performed. Intravascular ultrasonography was then performed, revealing patent TPT, proximal PT and peroneal arteries. Final angiographic images demonstrated brisk anterograde flow (Figure 50.6). The resting ABI increased to 0.84. At 3 years and 6 years after the intervention, there is sustained tissue integrity (Figures 50.7 and 50.8) and the ABI has remained at above 0.70.

Commentary

There are several important caveats with regard to infrapopliteal arterial disease that this case highlights: knee-to-foot patency of one of the three branches is

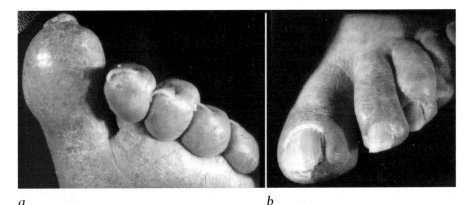

a   *b*

Figure 50.7 (a–b) *Appearance at 3 years of follow-up.*

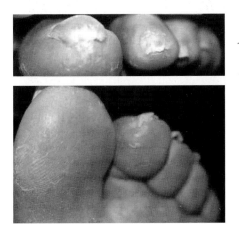

Figure 50.8 *(a–b) Appearance at 6 years of follow-up.*

a

b

211

usually sufficient to prevent critical lower-limb ischemia; claudication is rarely the result of isolated disease of the infrapopliteal arteries; re-stenosis after intervention in these vessels is typically the highest among the lower limb sites; and obstructive disease in these arteries is often occlusive, diffuse and complicated by heavy calcific deposits.

This case also underscores the typically difficult management decisions in the treatment of infrapopliteal disease. Importantly, no medical treatment has been shown to alter the natural history of critical limb ischemia and surgical revascularization procedures have several limitations in this group; there is a well-documented, short-lived patency of prosthetic materials used as conduits for lower-extremity distal bypass surgery. Furthermore, long-term patency of native vein (either as a reversed autologous graft or more frequently as an in situ graft) is still inferior to that reported for suprapopliteal disease, and in situ bypass surgery appears to have a higher risk of infectious complications than do most other lower-extremity vascular procedures.

At present, distal lower-extremity bypass surgery is primarily used for those patients with an advanced Rutherford (IV–VI) classification. However, in patients with Rutherford class IV (rest pain) or V (minor tissue loss), a percutaneous approach (if technically feasible) may have several advantages over reconstructive surgery, as exemplified in this presentation. It may defer surgical therapy, thus preserving native veins. It may accelerate healing of an ulcerative lesion or obviate superimposed infections or both. In more advanced cases, it may lower the anatomic level of proposed amputation and thereby preserve mobility by helping to heal a more limited (e.g. transmetatarsal) amputation site.

Uninterrupted patency of at least one of the three major infrapopliteal arteries is generally sufficient to expedite healing of a distal ulcerative lesion (see Figure 50.1). In patients in whom infrapopliteal disease coexists with SFA/popliteal disease, it is our practice to limit associated treatment of the infrapopliteal disease to short (< 2 cm) stenoses or occlusions or both. However, in patients with critical limb ischemia, limb salvage is paramount. Furthermore, the incidence of re-stenosis (which remains high in these patients irrespective of the technique used) should not be a factor in the decision to use a percutaneous approach: if uninterrupted patency of even one vessel can be achieved, improvement in antegrade nutrient flow is usually adequate to facilitate limb salvage. Once healed, most patients will do well, even in the face of documented re-stenosis, provided that they can avoid subsequent foot trauma.

References

1. European Working Group on Critical Leg Ischemia, Second European consensus document on chronic critical leg ischemia. *Circulation* 1991;**84**:IV-1–26.

2. Hallet JW, Jr., Brewster DC, Darling RC, The limitation of polytetrafluoroethylene in the reconstruction of femoropopliteal and tibial arteries. *Surg Gynecol Obstet* 1981;**152**:819–21.

3. Charlesworth PM, Brewster DC, Darling RC, Robison JG, Hallet JW, The fate of polytetrafluoroethylene grafts in lower limb bypass surgery: a six-year follow-up. *Br J Surg* 1985;**72**:896–9.

4. Veith FJ, Bupta SK, Ascer E et al, Six year prospective multicenter randomized comparison of autologous saphenous vein and expanded polytetrafluoroethyelene grafts in infrainguinal arterial reconstructions. *J Vasc Surg* 1986;**3**:104–14.

5. Leather RP, Shah DM, In situ saphenous vein arterial bypass. In: Rutherford RB, ed., *Vascular Surgery*, 3rd edn. Philadelphia: WB Saunders, 1992:422–30.

6. Reivsnyder T, Bandyk D, Seabrook G, Kinney E, Towne JB, Wound complications of the in situ saphenous vein bypass technique. *J Vasc Surg* 1992;**15**:843–8.

7. Miller N, Dardik H, Wolodiger F et al, Transmetatarsal amputation: the role of adjunctive revascularization. *J Vasc Surg* 1991;**13**:705–11.

213

Index